AMERICAN MEDICAL ASSOCIATION ESSENTIAL GUIDE TO HYPERTENSION

Whether you've just been diagnosed with hypertension or have been dealing with high blood pressure for a number of years, you can rely on the *American Medical Association Essential Guide to Hypertension* for clear, easy-to-understand answers to the many complex questions surrounding this chronic condition.

At least fifty million Americans have high blood pressure, but of them, as many as one-third may not be aware of their condition, as there are usually no obvious symptoms. The successful treatment of hypertension depends on knowledge—from recent medical advances that have improved blood pressure treatment to important steps you can take to help manage your blood pressure. This comprehensive guide begins with the basics of high blood pressure and its causes, and provides information on the latest medical research, breakthrough drug treatments, a healthy lifestyle, emergency situations, special needs and considerations for specific groups, hypertension and other diseases, and resources for locating additional help and information.

A member of the National High Blood Pressure Education Program, the American Medical Association strives to improve the health of people with hypertension through this indispensable guide.

American
Medical
Association

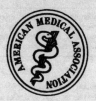

ESSENTIAL
GUIDE
TO
HYPERTENSION

POCKET BOOKS
New York   London   Toronto   Sydney   Singapore

The information, procedures, and recommendations in this book are not intended as a substitute for the medical advice of a trained health professional. All matters regarding your health require medical supervision. Consult your physician before adopting the suggestions in this book, as well as about any condition that may require diagnosis or medical attention.

In addition, statements made by the author regarding certain products do not constitute an endorsement of any product, service, or organization by the author or publisher, each of whom specifically disclaims any responsibility for any liability, loss, or risk, personal or otherwise, which is incurred as a consequence, directly or indirectly, of the use and application of any of the contents of this book or any of the products mentioned herein.

POCKET BOOKS, a division of Simon & Schuster Inc.
1230 Avenue of the Americas, New York, NY 10020

Copyright © 1998 by American Medical Association

Originally published in trade paperback in 1998 by Pocket Books

All rights reserved, including the right to reproduce
this book or portions thereof in any form whatsoever.
For information address Pocket Books, 1230 Avenue
of the Americas, New York, NY 10020

ISBN: 0-7434-0360-6

First Pocket Books mass market paperback printing April 2000

10 9 8 7 6 5 4 3

POCKET and colophon are registered trademarks of
Simon & Schuster Inc.

Cover design by Elizabeth Van Itallie
Cover photo by Michael Krasowitz/FPG International

Printed in the U.S.A.

American Medical Association

Physicians dedicated to the health of America

Foreword

You or a family member may be one of the more than 50 million Americans who have high blood pressure, or hypertension. Without treatment, hypertension can shorten your life by 10 to 20 years. The good news is that you can take relatively simple steps to manage your blood pressure and reduce your risk of developing life-threatening complications. The *American Medical Association Essential Guide to Hypertension* provides accurate, clear, up-to-date information to help you and your family deal effectively with hypertension.

This book describes hypertension, its possible causes, and how it can damage the body. It guides you through important lifestyle changes you can make, such as losing weight, modifying your diet, becoming more active, and reducing stress. This book will also help you understand the many different medications used to treat high blood pressure. Such information can help you work more effectively with your physician to control your blood pressure and to make informed decisions about your health care.

The member physicians of the AMA offer you this information as part of a continuing effort to help you and your family stay healthy. If you have access to the Internet, you can locate more health information by visiting the AMA website at **http://www.ama-assn.org**; if you need a doctor, you can access Physician Select: Online Doctor Finder, where you can search for information by specialty or by the doctor's name.

The American Medical Association wishes you and your family the best of health.

Nancy W. Dickey, MD
President, American Medical Association

The American Medical Association

Lynn E. Jensen, Chief Operating Officer
Robert L. Kennett, Senior Vice President,
    Publishing and Business Services
M. Frances Dyra, Director, Product Line Development

Editorial Staff

Angela Perry, MD, Medical Editor
Patricia Dragisic, Managing Editor
Steven Michaels, Senior Editor
Michelle Kienholz, Writer
Barbara Scotese, Editor
Laura M. Barnes, Editorial Assistant

Acknowledgments

Steven N. Blair, PED, Exercise/Fitness
Sheldon Berger, MD, Internal Medicine
Aleta Clark, MD, Pediatrics
Janis Donnaud, Literary Agent
Thomas Houston, MD, American Medical Association
Ramona Slupik, MD, Gynecology
Rolin Graphics, Inc., Minneapolis

Contents

Contents

Introduction

You probably purchased this book because you or someone you know has high blood pressure. You are not alone. At least 50 million Americans have high blood pressure. The medical term for this condition is *hypertension*. You probably would not describe yourself as "hyper" or "tense," though. You probably do not even have any symptoms—at least no symptoms that would suggest that you have a potentially life-threatening disorder. However, untreated hypertension may cut your life short by 10 to 20 years. And even if your blood pressure is not much above normal, you have an increased chance of damage to your heart, kidneys, eyes, or brain if high blood pressure is left untreated.

Since the 1970s, however, doctors have made a great deal of progress in the detection and treatment of high blood pressure. This progress has saved millions of lives and decreased the risk of health problems caused by hypertension. Some people can successfully manage their blood pressure with lifestyle changes only. If you are committed to maintaining healthy habits, you may never need to take any blood pressure medications. If you are not, though, you will need to take medication along with changing your lifestyle. You can then work with your doctor to determine the amount and type of medication you need to control your blood pressure.

In the *American Medical Association Essential Guide to Hypertension*, you will find all the information you will need to understand this common disorder and to manage your blood pressure safely and effectively. If you have just learned that you have high blood pressure, you may want to start at the beginning, learning the basics about how the body controls blood pressure, what can cause it to become elevated, and which health problems can result from uncontrolled hypertension. A glossary at the back of the book explains common medical terms related to hypertension and its treatment.

If you have had high blood pressure for many years, you will find here the latest information on monitoring your blood pressure, making lifestyle changes, and tailoring your drug therapy to match your personal needs. You can also catch up on what research has shown about hypertension in certain groups, such as women, blacks, older adults, children, and people with diabetes and other health problems. Finally, you will find answers to common questions and suggestions on where to go for help and additional information.

As a member of the National High Blood Pressure Education Program, the American Medical Association is committed to teaching people with hypertension how to live long, productive, enjoyable lives. We encourage you to use the information in this book to become a full partner with your doctor in the management of your blood pressure.

1

How Your Body Controls Blood Pressure

To understand why high blood pressure is a serious health problem, you first need to become familiar with the concept of blood pressure. This chapter reviews how and why the body maintains blood pressure and what can go wrong in the many systems involved.

Your heart and blood vessels work together to deliver oxygen and nutrients throughout the body and to remove waste products, such as the carbon dioxide you exhale with each breath. Blood is the medium through which these substances are transported. Blood pressure is the result of two opposing forces in the body: the force created by the heart when it pumps blood out and the force of the arteries (blood vessels that carry oxygen and nutrients to the tissues) as they resist this blood flow. The force generated by the heart when it contracts is called the systolic blood pressure; the force against the walls of the arteries when the heart relaxes is called the diastolic blood pressure. If the force of the heart pumping blood or of the arteries resisting blood flow (or both) are too great, you have hypertension.

A CARDIOVASCULAR PRIMER

You need oxygen and food to survive. Your body has a sophisticated method for delivering oxygen and nutrients to each of the millions of cells that make up your tissues and organs. Blood is kept in constant circulation by the pumping action of your heart. The heart sends blood first to the lungs to pick up oxygen, then to the rest of the body, and back to the heart through a system of tubes known as the vascular system. Because the heart and blood vessels (the vascular system) are all joined in one continuous and interdependent circuit, you will usually hear this called the cardiovascular system.

Your heart is the small, powerful pump that moves blood through the cardiovascular system. Even though it is not much larger than a clenched fist, your heart is the hardest working muscle in your body. Your heart beats approximately once each second and is responsible for pushing 10 to 11 pints of blood through 60,000 to 100,000 miles of blood vessels.

Your heart is divided into four chambers separated by valves that prevent backflow and intermingling of blood among the chambers. Blood that has circulated through the body is received by the first heart chamber, the right atrium. Once this oxygen-poor blood has been collected in the atrium, it is pushed into the

The heart

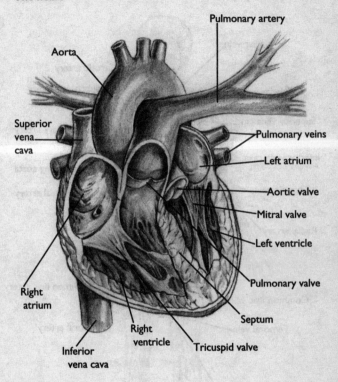

- Pulmonary artery
- Aorta
- Superior vena cava
- Pulmonary veins
- Left atrium
- Aortic valve
- Mitral valve
- Left ventricle
- Pulmonary valve
- Right atrium
- Septum
- Tricuspid valve
- Right ventricle
- Inferior vena cava

The circulatory system

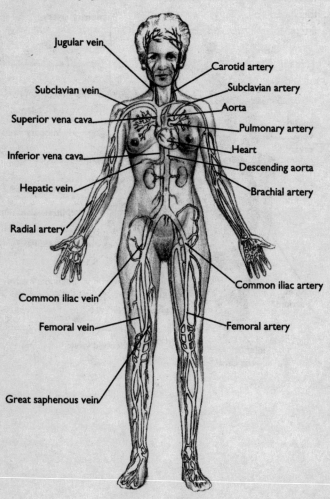

Jugular vein

Carotid artery

Subclavian vein

Subclavian artery

Superior vena cava

Aorta

Pulmonary artery

Inferior vena cava

Heart

Descending aorta

Hepatic vein

Brachial artery

Radial artery

Common iliac artery

Common iliac vein

Femoral vein

Femoral artery

Great saphenous vein

next heart chamber, the right ventricle. The right ventricle sends this "used" blood straight to the lungs through the pulmonary artery (the only artery to carry oxygen-poor blood). The lung tissues filter out the carbon dioxide and supply oxygen to the blood. This oxygen-rich blood returns to the next heart chamber, the left atrium, through the pulmonary veins (the only veins to carry oxygen-rich blood). When this oxygen-rich blood has collected in the left atrium, it is pushed into the final heart chamber, the left ventricle.

The left ventricle is the main pumping chamber of your heart. The largest and most powerful chamber, the left ventricle sends oxygen-rich blood through the aorta, the body's largest artery, to the entire body. The left ventricle works so hard that its muscular walls can be over one-half inch thick, more than three times thicker than those of the right ventricle.

Like any other organ, your heart needs oxygen and nutrients to function. The heart supplies blood to itself through two coronary arteries (right and left) that branch off the base of the aorta. The "used," oxygen-poor blood drains through the coronary veins directly into the right atrium. High blood pressure puts you at risk for coronary artery disease, so you can now see why these particular arteries are so important to keep healthy. When blood flow through these vessels is reduced or blocked, parts of your heart become weak and may even die. This is a heart attack.

So that it can separate the oxygen-rich blood from the "used" blood, the vascular system is divided into two components. Arteries deliver oxygen and nutrients from the heart to the body, and veins return oxygen-poor blood back to the heart, where the cycle begins again. Arteries and veins branch off into ever smaller and thinner walled vessels as they get farther from the heart and deeper into the tissues. The arterioles conduct blood from the arteries to the capillaries. Capillaries are the body's smallest blood vessels, which transmit oxygen and nutrients to individual cells and collect waste products. From the capillaries, blood low in oxygen and full of waste products flows first to venules (the smallest veins), which then pass blood along through veins back to the heart.

A healthy person's arteries are muscular and elastic. They stretch when the heart pumps blood through them. They can also change their diameter as needed to regulate the flow of blood. To raise blood pressure, the arterioles constrict or become narrow; to lower it, they dilate or widen. You will learn how and why in the sections ahead.

BLOOD PRESSURE CONTROL

You might think that your heart is responsible for your high blood pressure, but many organs and the chemicals they produce are involved. Because so many body systems are involved, researchers still have not determined the exact cause of hypertension. Blood pressure can be altered by anything that affects total cardiac output (the amount of blood your heart pumps) or total peripheral resistance (the degree to which blood vessels resist blood flow) or both.

Cardiac Output

Your heart, controlled by the brain, works to circulate blood continuously at a steady rate of about 5 quarts per minute. If you have excess fluid in your body, your blood volume goes up, causing both your cardiac output and your blood pressure to increase as well. The greater the volume of fluid, the harder your heart and blood vessels must work to circulate it. Diuretics, a common type of drug used to treat hypertension, work by reducing the volume of fluid in the body.

Your kidneys, the two bean-shaped organs in your lower back area, regulate the amount of fluid circulating in the body. They control fluid volume by either retaining salt and water or eliminating them in your urine. Normally, if you have eaten too much salt, your kidneys eliminate the excess sodium along with a certain amount of water. However, if your kidneys cannot get rid of the extra sodium, your body retains water, which raises blood volume and therefore blood pressure.

Two important chemicals are involved in maintaining the proper balance between sodium and water in the body. One is an enzyme produced by the kidney called renin. (Enzymes are proteins that speed up various chemical reactions in the body.) The kidney decides when to release renin on the basis of the amount of fluid in the body (which in turn is determined in part by the amount of salt you eat) and on the level of blood pressure in the arteries that supply the kidney. The lower the pressure, the more renin released. Renin acts by speeding up the conversion of angiotensinogen, another protein in the blood, to angiotensin. This reaction and its consequences are described in the next section.

Renin's by-products also stimulate the adrenal glands, which sit right on top of the kidneys, to produce a second chemical involved in regulating sodium levels in the body. This second chemical is a hormone called aldosterone. Unlike enzymes, hormones enter individual cells and serve as chemical messengers to their target tissues. Aldosterone goes from the adrenal glands into the blood and then to the kidneys. Aldosterone's chemical message to the kidneys is to retain more sodium and water. This retention of sodium and water elevates blood pressure.

The adrenal glands produce other hormones that affect cardiac output and blood pressure. When you are in a stressful situation of any sort, your brain preps the body for emergency action. One of the ways it does this is to send messages via the sympathetic nervous system to several organs. The sympathetic nervous system is one part of a larger portion of your nervous system, the autonomic nervous system. This system is responsible for controlling involuntary functions, such as breathing, digesting food, and controlling blood pressure.

When the adrenal glands receive an emergency signal from the sympathetic nervous system, they produce adrenaline or, as most doctors call it today, epinephrine, and noradrenaline (or norepinephrine). These hormones have several effects on the body. Epinephrine makes the heart beat faster. Norepinephrine is described in the next section. As you might expect, this sudden elevation in heart rate raises cardiac output and therefore blood pressure.

Peripheral Resistance

Your arteries play a more active role in regulating blood pressure than your heart does. The brain learns about fluctuations in blood pressure from special sensors in the walls of blood vessels that are part of the sympathetic nervous system. These baroreceptors, as they are called, notice when the pressure against the arterial wall goes up or down and relay this information to the brain. When your brain receives a signal that your blood pressure is too high, it sends a message through a collection of nerve cells (called vasomotor nerves) in your arteries to expand (or dilate) so blood can flow through more easily and under less pressure.

The brain also monitors the amount of oxygen and nutrients needed throughout the body. It adjusts blood pressure and blood flow to ensure that each organ's needs are being met. When the body is resting, the brain lowers blood pressure; when the body is under stress of any sort (including the stress of waking up), the brain raises blood pressure. The vasomotor nerves assist in accommodating these changes by telling the arteries to open (lowering blood pressure) or close (raising blood pressure).

As described above, the brain also readies the body for emergency situations by telling the adrenal glands to release epinephrine and norepinephrine. These hormones fit like keys into locks on specific tissues. These locks are called receptors, and when the hormone slips into them, it launches a certain action. Your heart has locks called beta receptors. When epinephrine and norepinephrine enter these receptors, your heart beats faster. Your kidneys also have beta receptors. When epinephrine and norepinephrine enter these receptors, the kidneys are stimulated to produce renin. You probably know of a type of high blood pressure drug called a beta blocker, which does exactly that: it fits into the beta receptor and blocks epinephrine and norepinephrine from triggering a rise in blood pressure.

Epinephrine and norepinephrine also fit into special locks on the arteries called alpha receptors. When this occurs, the artery constricts, raising blood pressure. Whether the walls of arteries and arterioles constrict depends on the amount of calcium inside the muscle cell. The constriction is triggered by a small amount of calcium passing into the cell through tiny passages called calcium channels. You may have heard about drugs called calcium channel blockers. These prevent the constriction of blood vessel walls by blocking the passage of calcium into the muscle cell. Drugs called alpha blockers work by preventing epinephrine and norepinephrine from triggering the constriction in the first place.

As mentioned in the last section, renin, an enzyme produced by the kidney (and other tissues in the body, such as the liver), is released when the body needs to raise blood pressure. However, renin does not directly affect blood pressure. Rather, it starts a chemical chain reaction by allowing one protein to convert into another, namely, angiotensinogen into angiotensin. If this angiotensin interacts with angiotensin converting enzyme (ACE—you have probably heard of ACE inhibitors, drugs that prevent this interaction), yet another substance is formed, called angiotensin II. Angiotensin II is an active chemical agent that causes arteries to contract and the adrenal glands to release aldosterone. The renin-angiotensin-aldosterone system is not completely understood yet, but research has shown that it is crucial to the development of high blood pressure. An even newer class of drugs called angiotensin blockers interfere with the action of this powerful chemical agent.

Many other factors affect resistance in the blood vessels. Too much fluid, besides increasing blood volume, makes tissues stiff. The arteries must contract harder to push blood into the tissues, so blood pressure goes up.

Blood pressure tends to rise with age because the arteries become harder and less flexible and thus put up more resistance to blood flow. The arteries in many people tend to become narrow and clogged with accumulated fatty debris over the years. This, too, raises blood pressure, owing to increased peripheral resistance. As you will learn in Chapters 2 and 6, smoking also causes the arteries to become stiffer and more resistant to blood flow.

WHAT IS HIGH BLOOD PRESSURE?

Although all these organs, nerve cells, and chemical messengers normally work together to maintain a healthy blood pressure, in some people something goes wrong that upsets this finely integrated system of checks and balances. Their blood pressure remains high even when the body does not need the additional force to distribute oxygen and nutrients. If the exact cause is unknown, doctors refer to the sustained high blood pressure as essential or primary hypertension, which is the most common type of high blood pressure. If the elevated blood pressure is caused by another disease or medication, doctors refer to it as secondary or disease-related hypertension.

Actually, there is no clear dividing line between normal and high blood pressure. The exact point at which sustained blood pressure is too high and can be classified as hypertension has instead been defined over the years on the basis of medical experience. Doctors have examined thousands of patients with different blood pressure levels and identified who was at highest risk for additional physical damage and disease. On the basis of many years of information, the Joint National Committee on Detection, Evaluation, and Treatment of High Blood Pressure established blood pressure guidelines to help Americans monitor their risk of hypertension and its unhealthy effects. How doctors diagnose and classify hypertension is described in Chapter 4.

2

Understanding Hypertension

For more than 95 percent of all people with hypertension, their condition has no identifiable cause. As we have said, this is called primary, or essential, hypertension. When you read about high blood pressure, essential hypertension is usually the type being discussed. Secondary hypertension is a potentially curable form of high blood pressure caused by an underlying disease or disorder.

HYPERTENSION IN THE US

Hypertension is the most common reason for visits to the doctor and for the use of prescription drugs in the US. As many as 50 million Americans have high blood pressure. Almost 40 percent of all blacks and more than half of all adults over age 60 (regardless of race) have hypertension. Of these, about 35 percent do not even know that they have high blood pressure. Only about half of all the people who are aware that they have hypertension are being treated.

In October 1995, representatives of eight professional medical groups released the first Hypertension Report Card on the Nation. The Hypertension Report Card gave an overall letter grade of C – to the detection, prevention, and treatment of hypertension in the US. Patient understanding of hypertension and communication between health-care professionals and patients both received a grade of D +. The 82 participants who developed the Hypertension Report Card included cardiologists, family physicians, internists, physician assistants, registered nurses, and members of the American Heart Association (AHA) Council for High Blood Pressure Research.

In a nation renowned for the quality of its health care, how can this be? For one thing, hypertension does not cause any obvious symptoms and may not be detected early. If left untreated, it can cause serious health problems and even death. Drugs used to treat high blood pressure can sometimes cause unpleasant side effects. Some people find these side effects especially bothersome and stop taking their medication on their own. And some people forget to take their medication every day. Others simply cannot afford their medication and may skip doses to try to make each refill last longer than it should. Some people do not fully understand the chronic nature of their hypertension and the need to make lifestyle changes, take medication as prescribed, and work closely with their doctor to manage the disease and prevent complications.

Despite these problems and thanks to new drugs, widespread screening, and increased public awareness, the incidence of hypertension in the US has declined since 1971: average systolic blood pressure has dropped from 131 to 119 mm Hg, and diastolic blood pressure has dropped from 83 to 73 mm Hg. (For an explanation of systolic and diastolic blood pressure, see page 47.)

WHO IS AT RISK FOR HYPERTENSION?

Essential hypertension tends to run in families. If your parents or siblings have high blood pressure, you may be more likely to develop the disease. As you learned in Chapter 1, many organ systems are involved in the regulation of blood pressure, and inherited problems in any of them could contribute to the development of hypertension.

Part of the reason that hypertension tends to run in families may be related to the fact that excess body weight tends to be a family characteristic, too. Studies suggest that 6 of every 10 adults with hypertension are 20 percent or more over their ideal body weight. If you are heavier than you should be, your blood pressure is likely to be higher than normal. In younger adults, the effect of weight on blood pressure is even more pronounced: risk of hypertension is 5 times higher in overweight people aged 20 to 44 but only twice as high in overweight people over 45. In a 5-year study of adults who started with normal or slightly elevated blood pressure, those who went on to develop hypertension were also very likely to be overweight. On the other hand, losing just 10 pounds can reduce your blood pressure.

In the fall of 1992, the AHA formally designated inactivity as one of the four top risk factors for the development of hypertension, heart attack, and stroke. Even if you are not overweight, being physically inactive can increase your likelihood of high blood pressure. Note that whether you are training at a gym, gardening, doing housework, jogging, or walking briskly, you are exercising your cardiovascular system, which helps it to work more efficiently and lower your blood pressure.

High blood pressure is almost twice as common in blacks as in whites. It affects more than one third of all African Americans and two thirds of those over age 60. Older black women have the highest incidence of hypertension. High blood pressure is the number-one preventable cause of more than 65,000 deaths annually among African Americans. Hypertension develops earlier in life in blacks than in whites (especially in women) and is usually more severe. African Americans have a higher rate of fatal stroke, fatal heart disease, and kidney failure related to their high blood pressure. In the US, black men living in high-stress areas (low income, high crime, and high unemployment) have been found to have higher blood pressure than those who live in less stressful environments.

As mentioned in Chapter 1, blood pressure usually goes up with age. This is particularly true for women. Before they reach menopause, women are less likely than men to have high blood pressure; after menopause, they are more likely to have high blood pressure. Among older adults, blood pressure rises because of the accumulated effects of deteriorating flexibility and strength in the arteries, increasing amounts of blockage in the arteries, reduced ability of the body to maintain a healthy balance of sodium and fluid, and a lower level of physical activity and overall fitness. Older adults are also more likely to have other health problems, such as diabetes or high cholesterol levels. They often take one or more medications daily, some of which can raise blood pressure. Finally, many older adults have high systolic blood pressure but normal diastolic pressure, which they may not recognize as serious.

Smoking is connected with so many serious health problems that you probably will not be surprised to learn that it can put you at risk for high blood pressure. Chemicals in tobacco smoke injure the delicate lining of arteries and make them more susceptible to blockage. And nicotine is a powerful stimulant that affects the nerves that regulate the heart and blood vessels. As described in Chapter 1, when these nerves are stimulated, heart rate goes up, arteries contract, and blood pressure rises. Smoking is also associated with an increase in the amount of total and low density lipoprotein (LDL, or "bad") cholesterol in your blood (both of which contribute to blockages in the arteries) and a decrease in the amount of high density lipoprotein (HDL, or "good") cholesterol.

Using even smokeless tobacco can put you at risk for hypertension. Smokeless tobacco contains nicotine, sodium, and licorice, all of which raise blood pressure. The typical nicotine exposure from smokeless tobacco is greater than that from smoking an average cigarette. Sodium content per serving ranges from 200 to 1,200 milligrams. (Doctors recommend that people take in no more than 2,400 milligrams of sodium per day.) Natural licorice, as you will read later in this chapter, can raise blood pressure by causing the body to retain sodium.

Drinking can also result in hypertension, particularly if you consume large amounts of alcohol. In a study of more than 80,000 adults, a slight increase in blood pressure occurred in men who had 1 to 2 drinks per day; in women, an increase was noted in those who had 3 or more drinks per day. One drink (12 ounces of beer, 4 ounces of wine, or 1.25 ounces of 86-proof whiskey) contains about 13 grams of alcohol, and research shows that blood pressure goes up steadily if you drink more than 20 to 24 grams of alcohol per day. The type of alcoholic beverage is irrelevant.

Finally, many people associate stress with high blood pressure. Stress is an imbalance between physical or mental demands and your body's ability to cope with them. As described in Chapter 1, a stressful situation triggers several chemical changes in the body. An increase in high blood pressure is one result of these chemical changes. Usually, the elevated blood pressure is temporary and returns to normal after the stressful situation has passed. While stress may contribute to high blood pressure in some people, the nature of the connection between stress and hypertension is still under investigation.

ESSENTIAL HYPERTENSION

In 95 percent of people with hypertension, the cause is unknown and therefore not specifically treatable. Considerable evidence suggests that hypertension may result from a problem in the kidneys. Studies of kidney transplantations reveal that a kidney donated by someone with hypertension can cause hypertension in the recipient, and that a kidney donated by someone with normal blood pressure can eliminate existing hypertension in the recipient. Researchers believe that slight changes in kidney function early in life are important in the later development of hypertension.

Doctors now realize that the bodies of people with essential hypertension may respond differently to treatment owing to individual differences in their kidney function. For example, about one in five people with essential hypertension has kidneys that do not produce much renin. This is more common in blacks than in whites. A slightly smaller percentage of people with essential hypertension produce too much renin. More than one fourth of people with essential hypertension seem to have problems in their adrenal glands and their kidneys that prevent the body from properly regulating sodium levels. All of these differences are important because they affect how people's bodies respond to treatment.

TREATABLE CAUSES OF HYPERTENSION

For a small number of people with hypertension, there is a known—and potentially curable—cause for their high blood pressure. This form of the disease is known as secondary hypertension, because the increase in blood pressure is secondary to (caused by) an underlying disease or disorder.

If you are wondering whether you have secondary hypertension, you might consider whether any of these characteristics apply to you:

- Secondary hypertension often comes on suddenly and without warning.
- Secondary hypertension is usually the cause of high blood pressure in children.

- Secondary hypertension usually produces very high blood pressure readings.
- Secondary hypertension is associated with wide swings in blood pressure.
- Secondary hypertension is often accompanied by other unusual symptoms that lead to the discovery of the problem.

Tests to diagnose secondary hypertension are discussed in Chapter 4. In most cases, doctors treat the underlying cause itself. If the underlying disease or disorder can be cured, blood pressure usually returns to normal.

In Chapter 1, you learned about the various body systems involved in regulating blood pressure. Not surprisingly, defects or diseases in these organs can reduce their ability to help maintain normal blood pressure. The most common disorders are described below.

Kidneys

Because the kidneys play such an important role in the regulation of blood pressure, certain diseases of the kidney can cause hypertension. In fact, about 3 percent to 4 percent of all cases of hypertension are related to kidney problems. This is especially true in younger people and people who have diabetes. Simple urine tests can often be used to identify hypertension caused by kidney disorders.

RENOVASCULAR HYPERTENSION

Renovascular hypertension is the most common form of secondary hypertension. It occurs when the arteries that supply the kidneys with blood (the renal arteries) become mostly (more than half) or fully blocked. If the blood supply to a kidney is reduced, the affected kidney responds by releasing renin. As you learned in Chapter 1, renin raises blood pressure not only within the renal arteries but throughout the body.

In most people with renovascular hypertension, the arteries are blocked with plaques (explained in Chapter 3). In some cases, the renal arteries can be bypassed completely with surgery or the blockage can be relieved with a balloon catheter (angioplasty). Once the artery is open again, blood pressure usually returns to normal. People with this type of renovascular hypertension tend to be older (above 55 years old) and to have higher systolic blood pressure. They are also more likely to have blocked arteries elsewhere in their body, such as the coronary arteries (which supply the heart with blood) or the carotid arteries (which supply the brain with blood).

FIBROMUSCULAR HYPERPLASIA

Renovascular hypertension can also be caused by fibromuscular hyperplasia. In this disorder, the muscle and fibrous tissues of the renal arteries (the arteries that supply the kidneys with blood) increase in bulk and harden into rings. Like the more common atherosclerotic plaques, these rings of fibrous tissue block the flow of blood through the renal arteries. Fibromuscular hyperplasia occurs mainly in young white women (usually before age 30) and may be aggravated by pregnancy. The renal arteries can be bypassed with surgery or widened with a balloon catheter (angioplasty), allowing blood pressure to return to normal.

GLOMERULONEPHRITIS

Your kidneys are responsible for filtering out and eliminating waste products and excessive amounts of other substances in the body, such as sodium. The tiny filtering units in the kidneys are called glomeruli. Glomerulonephritis is the inflammation of these filters. The inflamed glomeruli cannot function properly and eventually may become permanently damaged and fail. As a result, blood pressure goes up significantly. If glomerulonephritis comes on suddenly, such as in response to an infection, the urine is dark (often bloody), and the severely elevated blood pressure can cause headaches and vision problems. Acute (sudden) glomerulonephritis occurs most often in children and young adults. Chronic glomerulonephritis begins gradually and continues over many years. Symptoms are much less obvious in chronic glomerulonephritis until the kidneys have been seriously damaged by the disease. Treatment depends on the form of the disease you have, and many milder cases of acute glomerulonephritis may clear up on their own. In acute cases the underlying cause is treated. In both chronic and acute cases, treatment for high blood pressure includes antihypertensive drugs.

POLYCYSTIC KIDNEY DISEASE

Polycystic kidney disease is an inherited disorder in which many cysts (fluid-filled lumps) in both kidneys cause an increase in size and a decrease in function. The cysts can be detected in fetuses with the aid of an ultrasound scan or genetic testing during pregnancy, or the disease can go undetected until later in childhood, when symptoms such as multiple urinary tract infections and blood in the urine may occur. The cysts can interfere with normal kidney function, causing urinary tract infections and hypertension, both of which must be treated as needed with appropriate drugs. Polycystic kidney disease can be treated only through kidney transplantation.

HYDRONEPHROSIS

Hydronephrosis occurs when certain areas of the kidney become inflamed and urine flow is blocked. Hydronephrosis can come on suddenly or gradually, can occur in one or both kidneys, and can result from congenital (present from birth) obstruction. The resulting damage to kidney tissue can cause elevated blood pressure. Surgery is required to drain excess fluid and correct the blockage. Once the kidneys are functioning normally again, blood pressure usually returns to normal levels.

Adrenal and Other Glands

The adrenal glands are located on top of the kidneys. Anything that interferes with the normal function of the adrenal glands may also raise blood pressure. Disorders in other glands in the body, such as the pituitary gland (in the brain), the thyroid gland (in the neck), and the parathyroid glands (in the neck), can also affect blood pressure.

ALDOSTERONISM

Aldosterone is a hormone produced by the adrenal glands. It regulates the balance of sodium and potassium in the blood, indirectly affecting blood pressure. A tumor in the adrenal gland can cause it to produce too much aldosterone, resulting in a condition known as aldosteronism. Disorders elsewhere in the body, such as heart failure, cirrhosis of the liver, and kidney disease, can also trigger excessive aldosterone production. As explained in Chapter 1, too much aldosterone will force the kidneys to retain too much salt, thereby leading to high blood pressure. Hypertension caused by aldosteronism is usually accompanied by muscle weakness, excessive urination or thirst, and too little potassium in the blood. Low blood potassium levels are an important diagnostic clue to these rare tumors, as is a low or normal associated renin level. If only one adrenal gland is affected, a surgeon can remove it. If both adrenal glands are involved and several small tumors have developed, drug treatment is required to block the effects of aldosterone. Finally, if the aldosteronism is caused by another disorder in the body, that disease must be treated before aldosterone levels (and blood pressure) will return to normal.

PHEOCHROMOCYTOMA

Epinephrine (also called adrenaline) is a hormone produced by the adrenal glands. Among other things, it is involved in the regulation of heart rate and blood flow. An abnormality, such as a tumor, can cause the adrenal glands to produce too much epinephrine. This excess production of epinephrine may be sustained or may occur in spurts and cause such symptoms as high blood pressure, a pounding heartbeat, headache, sweating, anxiety, and trembling. This condition is known as pheochromocytoma. Between bouts, the person generally feels normal and may have normal blood pressure. Sometimes, however, pheochromocytoma causes persistent (rather than intermittent) hypertension. In these cases, the person has usually lost weight and can have fever, headache, and persistently elevated blood pressure. Usually, the tumors that cause pheochromocytoma are benign (noncancerous) and can be surgically removed, restoring the person's blood pressure to normal levels.

CUSHING'S SYNDROME

The adrenal glands may also produce too much of another hormone called cortisol. This condition is known as Cushing's syndrome and it is treated mainly by endocrinologists (internists who are gland specialists). In addition to causing elevated blood pressure, the excess cortisol causes a rounded face, weight gain on the body (but not the limbs), weakness, bruising (purple stretch marks on the abdomen are common), and menstrual irregularity. A tumor in the pituitary gland (which controls the activity of the adrenal glands) may cause this syndrome. Sometimes an abnormal increase in the size of the adrenal glands (hyperplasia) or small tumors are the cause. Depending on the cause, treatment with surgery, radiation therapy, or drug therapy brings cortisol levels (and blood pressure) back to normal.

CONGENITAL ADRENAL HYPERPLASIA

Cortisol is a hormone produced by the adrenal glands. If cortisol cannot be made in a developing fetus, the adrenal glands produce large amounts of sex hormones and other chemical substances. This can cause any of several disorders that are collectively known as congenital adrenal hyperplasia. (*Congenital* means "from birth," and *hyperplasia* refers to an abnormal increase in the size of an organ—in this case, the adrenal glands.) The exact effects on the infant depend on when in the pregnancy the disorder began. Both sexes experience abnormal development of sexual organs. In some newborns, the adrenal glands fail immediately after birth. Fortunately, treatment with hydrocortisone stops the disorder and allows the baby to grow and develop normally.

HYPOTHYROIDISM

Also called myxedema, hypothyroidism occurs when the thyroid gland (located in your neck) stops functioning, slowing metabolism. Changes in facial appearance (puffiness), voice (hoarseness, slow speech), and hair and skin (coarseness, dryness, and scaliness) occur slowly. Other symptoms that gradually appear may include weight gain, memory loss, constipation, menstrual irregularity, and low body temperature. Primary (cause unknown) hypothyroidism is the most common form of this disorder, though radiation therapy, surgery, certain drugs, and problems with the pituitary gland can also affect thyroid function. Hypothyroidism, whatever the cause, is treated with hormone replacement therapy.

HYPERTHYROIDISM

Hyperthyroidism, the excessive production of hormones by the thyroid gland, occurs in Graves' disease, goiter, and several other disorders. One outcome of hyperthyroidism is an increase in adrenergic activity (that is, activity of the hormones epinephrine and norepinephrine, as explained in Chapter 1), which can cause a rise in blood pressure. Possible symptoms include weight loss, increased appetite, increased sweating, and insensitivity to cold. Rapid heart rate and tremors may also occur. Depending on the cause of the hyperthyroidism, treatment may involve the use of radioactive iodine, medication (including beta blockers, described in Chapter 8), or surgery.

ACROMEGALY

A rare hormonal problem known as acromegaly results from a certain type of tumor inside the pituitary gland (located in the brain). In this disorder, the pituitary gland produces too much growth hormone, which causes the facial bones, hands, and feet to grow larger than normal and swell. Many other organs, including the heart, become enlarged, and hypertension can also result. Surgery and radiotherapy are used to eliminate the tumor in the pituitary gland, and sometimes drugs are needed to lower growth hormone levels. Once acromegaly is successfully treated, blood pressure returns to normal.

HYPERPARATHYROIDISM

Another set of glands, the parathyroid glands, regulates calcium balance in the body. If the parathyroid glands become overactive (a condition known as primary hyperparathyroidism), they can cause blood pressure to rise. One possible result of hyperparathyroidism is kidney damage due to excessively high and sustained levels of calcium in the blood (a condition known as hypercalcemia). Other symptoms of the disorder include bone loss, constipation, nausea and vomiting, and frequent urination. The diseased portion of parathyroid gland is removed surgically to allow blood levels of calcium—and blood pressure—to drop to normal levels.

Arteries

As discussed earlier in this section, narrowing of the renal arteries can increase blood pressure. Major arteries throughout your body play a significant role in determining your blood pressure, and disorders within them can result in hypertension.

COARCTATION OF THE AORTA

If the body's main artery, the aorta, is unusually narrow, the blood supply to the kidneys is diminished. The kidneys respond by releasing renin (see Chapter 1) to raise blood pressure. This congenital (from birth) condition is known as coarctation of the aorta and usually requires corrective surgery.

AORTIC REGURGITATION

When the valves of the aorta (the body's main artery) cannot close tightly, blood flows back into the left ventricle of the heart. This is known as aortic regurgitation or aortic insufficiency. Because the left ventricle has more blood to pump back out to the body, systolic blood pressure is elevated. In addition, systolic blood pressure is considerably higher in the legs than in the arms. This isolated systolic hypertension ends when the cause of the valvular insufficiency is repaired, usually with surgery.

Medication

There is a list of types of medication that can raise blood pressure on page 30. Hypertension frequently occurs during use of oral contraceptives, cyclosporine (used by patients receiving organ transplants), and prescription and nonprescription drugs that contain sympathomimetics (chemicals that mimic the action of the sympathetic nervous system, including raising blood pressure) or glucocorticoids (compounds that reduce inflammation).

Nonsteroidal anti-inflammatory drugs (NSAIDs)—such as aspirin, ibuprofen, or naproxen sodium, and many other similar drugs used for general pain relief and arthritis treatment—can cause edema (fluid retention) and kidney problems, which can in turn raise blood pressure. Anti-inflammatory drugs that contain corticosteroids (such as cortisone and hydrocortisone) can also raise blood pressure. Appetite suppressants, antihistamines, and cold preparations that contain phentermine, methamphetamine, pseudoephedrine, or phenylpropanolamine also have hypertensive effects, particularly in people who already have high blood pressure.

MEDICATIONS THAT CAN CAUSE OR AGGRAVATE HYPERTENSION

Antidepressants (monoamine oxidase [MAO] inhibitors and tricyclics)
Anti-inflammatory drugs
Appetite suppressants
Cold remedies
Cyclosporine
Nasal decongestants

- Oxymetazoline
- Phenylephrine
- Phenylpropanolamine
- Pseudoephedrine

Nonsteroidal anti-inflammatory drugs (NSAIDs)

- Aspirin
- Ibuprofen
- Naproxen sodium

Oral contraceptives

Certain types of antidepressant medication, known as monoamine oxidase (MAO) inhibitors, can cause a hypertensive crisis that can be life-threatening. Tricyclic (this refers to the chemical structure of these drugs) antidepressant drugs can also raise blood pressure or interfere with antihypertensive medication.

Finally, some illegal drugs, especially cocaine and amphetamines, can raise blood pressure significantly.

Other Secondary Causes

There are other relatively rare or specialized causes of hypertension. Some causes of temporary elevation in blood pressure are reviewed elsewhere in this book. For example, heavy alcohol consumption can raise blood pressure significantly, as mentioned earlier in this chapter and discussed in more detail in Chapter 6. Secondary hypertension can also occur during pregnancy (see Chapter 12). In such cases, blood pressure may return to normal shortly after birth, or hypertension may persist, requiring lifelong treatment (as essential hypertension).

Consuming excessive amounts of the herb licorice (pure natural licorice used by practitioners of herbal medicine, not artificially flavored candies) can promote sodium retention and, in turn, hypertension. This is because natural licorice contains a chemical known as glycyrrhizic acid, a compound very similar to aldosterone, a hormone involved in regulating blood pressure (see Aldosteronism, page 24).

Some neurologic disorders are associated with elevated or unstable blood pressure. Guillain-Barré syndrome, which is charac-

---

YOU MAY BE AT RISK FOR HIGH BLOOD PRESSURE IF YOU . . .

- Have family members (parents, grandparents, brothers, sisters) with high blood pressure
- Are African American
- Are a man over age 35
- Are a woman over age 50 (or past menopause)
- Are overweight
- Smoke cigarettes or use smokeless tobacco
- Drink more than two or three alcoholic beverages per day on a regular basis
- Use oral contraceptives
- Do not exercise regularly

---

terized by sudden, rapid muscular weakness and sensory loss, can also cause fluctuations in blood pressure because of the disease's effect on the autonomic nervous system (see Chapter 1). In fact, any neurologic condition that affects the autonomic nervous system can also affect blood pressure. Elevated intracranial pressure (pressure on the brain), most often caused by head injuries, will also cause an increase in blood pressure.

3

How Hypertension Hurts Your Body

Hypertension is called "the silent killer" because it produces no obvious symptoms until serious damage has already occurred. If left uncontrolled, high blood pressure will damage the heart, arteries, kidneys, and brain. The eyes are also very sensitive to the effects of hypertension. People who experience large fluctuations in daily blood pressure—that is, much higher during the day than at night—are more likely to develop health problems related to their hypertension.

Research suggests that compared with people who have normal blood pressure, those who have uncontrolled hypertension may be three times more likely to develop coronary heart disease, six times more likely to develop congestive heart failure, and seven times more likely to have a stroke. However, none of the adverse effects described in this chapter are inevitable. You can prevent all health problems associated with hypertension by working closely with your doctor to control your blood pressure.

HEART

As the organ responsible for pumping blood throughout the body, your heart will eventually develop problems related to the strain of working against elevated pressure in the blood vessels. Like any muscle, the heart becomes enlarged when forced to work harder. The walls become thickened and shorter, causing the muscle to lose its full range of motion. Often, there is not enough blood to supply the enlarged heart with sufficient oxygen and nutrients. An enlarged heart is also more susceptible to irregular beats, known as arrhythmia, which feel like missed or extra beats.

When the largest chamber in your heart, the left ventricle (see Chapter 1), becomes abnormally enlarged, a condition known as left ventricular hypertrophy is diagnosed. As the wall thickens, it becomes more difficult for the ventricle to expand and therefore to fill completely with blood. Less and less blood is pumped out, leading to breathlessness, angina (chest pain), palpitations, and feeling faint. Blood may back up into blood vessels in the lungs, putting more pressure on these vessels and causing shortness of breath. If this process continues and the pressure gets very high, pulmonary edema, a flooding of the lungs with fluid, can result. Pulmonary edema, which causes severe shortness of breath, is a medical emergency and is potentially fatal if not treated quickly.

Your heart will also eventually begin to fail after many years of uncontrolled high blood pressure. When this happens, fluid from the blood again backs up in the lungs (making you feel congested). Muscles in the rest of the body become weak from a lack of oxygen, which is no longer adequately circulated by the failing heart. This is known as congestive heart failure. A person with congestive heart failure will have difficulty breathing during physical exertion early in the disease but will eventually feel short of breath all the time. Breathing becomes easier when the person sits in an upright position. In addition, other tissues become waterlogged—a condition known as edema—causing the feet and legs to swell with excess fluid.

In one large study that has been ongoing since the late 1940s, the Framingham Heart Study, doctors found that hypertension was responsible for almost 40 percent of the reported cases of congestive heart failure in men and almost 60 percent of the cases in women. Hypertension was previously diagnosed in 91 percent of the participants with congestive heart failure. The risk of developing congestive heart failure was twice as high in men and three times as high in women who had high blood pressure compared with those who had normal blood pressure levels. Less than one quarter of the men and less than one third of the women lived more than 5 years after being diagnosed with congestive heart failure.

The blood vessels responsible for supplying oxygen and energy to the heart, the coronary arteries, can also be damaged by high blood pressure. When the coronary arteries do not supply enough oxygen for your heart, you may experience pain, tightness, or heaviness in the chest for short periods during exertion. This is known as angina pectoris or, more commonly, angina. As with congestive heart failure, the effects of angina are felt during activity early in the disease but later come on more frequently, even at rest or during emotional situations.

Angina alone does not damage the heart but can serve as a warning of an impending heart attack (see the list of warning signs below). The pain of a heart attack lasts longer than angina and is usually accompanied by other symptoms, such as nausea and sweating. During a heart attack, blood is cut off from part of the heart because of a blockage in a coronary artery. The lack of blood causes this area of heart muscle to die. If a sufficiently large portion of the heart is deprived of blood, the heart will stop beating unless emergency health care is provided.

Left ventricular hypertrophy can also cause angina. The thickened muscle of the left ventricle squeezes small blood vessels until they have completely collapsed. Tissue nourished by these vessels may be deprived of oxygen for a short time, and the pain of angina may result. If your hypertension remains uncontrolled, left

---

Warning: The following symptoms may mean that you are having a heart attack:

- Crushing chest pain or pressure
- Chest pain that moves to your neck, jaw, arms, shoulders, or upper abdomen
- Dizziness
- Chills
- Heavy sweating
- Nausea and vomiting
- Severe shortness of breath
- Feeling extremely weak or fainting

Never ignore these symptoms. If you think that you may be having a heart attack, call **immediately** for emergency medical assistance or have someone take you directly to the nearest hospital emergency department.

---

ventricular hypertrophy will progress to a thinning of the heart muscle (due to tissue death caused by this loss of blood vessels). The heart loses much of its pumping power. This leads to congestive heart failure, when the heart can no longer circulate blood throughout the body, and, in some cases, end-stage heart disease.

ARTERIES

Your blood vessels can be damaged by high blood pressure. The force of the blood's pushing hard through your arteries can shear or tear off cells from the inside lining. Damaged arteries may repair themselves, but when the damage is extensive or occurs frequently, the repair process leads to a bulging plaque made of fat, cholesterol, and dead cells. People with elevated blood cholesterol levels, especially low density lipoprotein (LDL, or "bad") cholesterol, are at greatest risk for developing these fatty plaques. Hypertension accelerates the process, and the plaques can grow to a size that blocks the passage of blood. This process is known as atherosclerosis (see Atherosclerosis Explained, page 38), which can begin as early as childhood and continue for decades. Like hypertension, atherosclerosis is silent until sufficient damage has been done to cause symptoms. For almost one of every five people with atherosclerosis, a fatal heart attack is the first and only symptom.

Besides accelerating the blockage of arteries, high blood pressure can speed up arteriosclerosis (hardening of the arteries). This occurs when the muscles in your blood vessels become thickened and hard, narrowing the arteries and making them less flexible.

ATHEROSCLEROSIS EXPLAINED

Hypertension accelerates the process of atherosclerosis (see illustration) by creating areas of injured tissue along the inside lining of your arteries. When your blood pressure is high, the extra force of blood pounding against the delicate lining shears off cells, causing damage to the lining. Your arteries may also be damaged by harmful chemicals in cigarette smoke and by oxidized (chemically modified) low density lipoprotein (LDL, or "bad") cholesterol. You can reduce the amount of oxidized LDL in your blood by eating a diet rich in antioxidant vitamins—especially vitamins A, C, and E—which includes such foods as citrus fruits, leafy green vegetables, whole grains, and low-fat dairy products.

The damaged arterial walls attract white blood cells called monocytes. These are the type of white blood cells that attack bacteria and other foreign bodies in your blood. The monocytes attach to the damaged area to do their work and eventually burrow under the inside lining of the artery.

Once inside the arterial wall, the monocytes change into another type of cell called a macrophage, a cell that acts as a scavenger or "garbage collector" for the body. Macrophages eat dead cells to get them out of the way, and they also absorb LDL cholesterol. The macrophages in your arterial walls cannot be removed by blood flow for recycling, so they remain there permanently. When LDL in the blood finds its way into the damaged area of the artery, the macrophages absorb it and swell up into what is called a foam cell. If you have elevated levels of LDL in your blood, the LDL is more likely to enter these damaged areas and cause the macrophages to grow into foam cells. When several foam cells gather in one spot, a fatty streak (known as plaque) develops in the artery wall.

As the foam cells continue to grow, they push out against the lining of the artery, making the damaged area larger and interfering with blood flow. The additional damage to the artery attracts another type of blood cell called a platelet. Platelets stick to the damaged site and release a chemical that encourages the delicate arterial lining to grow back. Smooth muscle in the artery wall also grows in response to this chemical. With this accumulation of cells and extra growth of tissue, the artery gradually becomes more and more narrow—and sometimes completely blocked.

The clumping of platelets at the damaged site adds to the risk as the clot collects calcium, fibrous tissue, and other debris in the blood. The clot could then break loose, especially under the extra force of high blood pressure, and block an artery, possibly causing a stroke or heart attack.

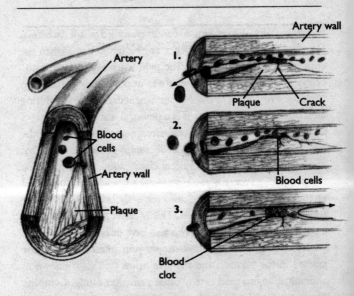

Plaque buildup in the artery wall can cause a blood clot to form. **1.** Cracks appear in the surface of the plaque. **2.** The body reacts as though the cracks are an injury, and begins to form a blood clot around them. **3.** The clot grows and blocks blood flow.

The result is the same: less blood passes through the vessels to the tissues.

When narrowing occurs in the arteries that supply your heart with blood (usually due to buildup of plaques), you develop coronary artery disease. Ischemic heart disease (ischemic refers to obstruction of the blood supply) occurs as a result of atherosclerosis in the coronary arteries, or constriction of the coronary arteries caused by spasm (involuntary contraction of the muscles in the artery walls). Occasionally, such narrowing can occur without producing any discomfort, a condition called silent ischemia. However, most people experience angina (chest pain) when tissues are deprived of oxygen. The pain is usually located in the center of the chest but may radiate to or occur only in the neck, shoulder, arm, or lower jaw. No permanent damage occurs during an angina attack, but, again, it is a powerful warning sign.

A blockage in an artery can damage any body part. In the legs, narrowed arteries cause pain or cramps while you walk. This condition is known as intermittent claudication. As with angina, the pain will go away if you rest. However, severe and untreated arterial blockage in the legs can eventually cause tissues in the toes (and on up the legs) to die. This is called gangrene, which is a special concern for people who also have diabetes.

Narrowing of arteries that supply your intestines can cause cramps in the stomach and the area below it. This is known as abdominal angina, and it may cause pain after eating. Complete blockage of a blood vessel to the intestines can cause blood to appear in the stools and, eventually, that portion of the intestine may die. If the intestine perforates, bacteria can leak into the abdomen, causing infection of the abdomen (peritonitis) or death.

With blocked arteries, there is also the risk that pieces of the blockage (plaque) may break off and travel in the bloodstream. If some of this plaque becomes stuck in a blood vessel and blocks blood flow, tissues beyond that point will begin to die. In the heart, this is known as a heart attack; in the brain, as a stroke.

If blood pressure is severely elevated, the risks can be even more serious. Rather than gradually narrowing the arteries, very high blood pressure can cause a weakened blood vessel to burst. The released blood seriously damages the surrounding tissues. In the brain, a stroke of this type is often fatal. The largest artery in the body, the aorta, may develop a bulge due to very high blood pressure. This bulge is known as an aneurysm, and such aneurysms may burst. However, these potentially deadly effects of severely elevated blood pressure may be accompanied by warning symptoms: headache, dizziness, nosebleeds, blurred vision, and sometimes chest or abdominal pain.

KIDNEYS

Because your kidneys must filter all the blood in your body, they are very susceptible to damage by uncontrolled hypertension. Each of the damaging effects to blood vessels discussed above also applies to the renal arteries (arteries that supply the kidneys). As discussed in Chapter 2, narrowing of the renal arteries can cause renovascular hypertension, which can be corrected with surgery to open the arteries.

Kidney tissue itself may eventually become damaged by severe high blood pressure. The ability of this tissue to filter out waste products gradually declines until it fails. Waste products build up as toxins (poisons) in the blood in a condition known as uremia. Early symptoms of kidney failure include fatigue, inability to concentrate, and muscle cramps. Without early treatment, nausea, vomiting, gastrointestinal bleeding, an unpleasant taste in the mouth, and loss of appetite eventually occur. People whose kidneys fail must undergo a procedure called dialysis, which filters waste from the blood. While some people may fear that drugs prescribed to control blood pressure may damage their kidneys, medication is essential for preserving kidney function.

When the small arteries and arterioles of the kidney become

hardened and blocked, the condition is known as nephrosclerosis. Benign nephrosclerosis is a gradual and prolonged deterioration of these vessels in which the inner layer of the walls of smaller arteries thickens. Fat is then deposited in the degenerated wall tissue until the channel becomes blocked. Malignant nephrosclerosis occurs at a much faster rate, causing hemorrhage (bleeding into the tissues), ruptures, and swollen tissues. The symptoms of nephrosclerosis include impaired vision, blood in the urine, weight loss, and uremia. Treatment includes antihypertensive drugs, elimination of infection and blockage, and other measures for relief of chronic kidney failure, such as dialysis. Progressive kidney failure is associated with all stages of hypertension but is much more common in people with stages 2, 3, and 4 (see Chapter 4).

BRAIN

Arteries supplying blood to your brain can experience similar damage as that described above because of chronic high blood pressure. The vessels may thicken and become narrow, or a clot may form, blocking blood flow to a specific part of the brain. A clot that forms in the brain is called a cerebral thrombosis and causes one type of stroke. Depending on which blood vessels are affected, a person who has a stroke may lose the ability to speak, walk, or move one side of the body. A clot that breaks away from a blood vessel elsewhere in the body, such as the carotid arteries (the large arteries in the neck that supply blood to the brain), and lodges in a brain blood vessel is known as a cerebral embolus.

In addition, one or more bulges can develop in the arteries

inside the brain. These are known as cerebral aneurysms, which may eventually burst, causing bleeding in the brain (cerebral hemorrhage). This is another type of stroke, one that usually causes more damage than cerebral thrombosis. A stroke due to cerebral hemorrhage is more likely to result in death than one due to a clot.

Of the estimated 500,000 Americans who have strokes each year, about 25 percent to 30 percent die, making stroke the third most common cause of death in the US. Even when strokes are not fatal, they are often debilitating: stroke is the number-one cause of disability among older adults in the US. Strokes can cause paralysis, speech loss, hearing loss, blindness, memory loss, and many other devastating effects.

About 70 percent to 80 percent of people who have strokes also have hypertension. Evidence suggests that a person with untreated hypertension is almost seven times more likely to have a stroke than a person with normal blood pressure or controlled hypertension. Even high normal and mild hypertension contribute significantly to stroke risk. Controlling blood pressure is the best preventive measure to take to reduce the risk of stroke. Other preventive steps include not smoking, eating less saturated fat, becoming more physically active, and taking low-dose (children's) aspirin.

One of the few warning signs of stroke is a so-called ministroke or transient ischemic attack (TIA). Unlike a full-blown stroke, in which damage to the brain is permanent, a ministroke produces strokelike symptoms that last from a few minutes to several hours and disappear within 24 hours. Symptoms may include sudden weakness, clumsiness, or numbness in one arm, leg, or side of the face. Loss of vision, double vision, and an inability to speak or to speak coherently may also occur. If you experience a TIA, you should talk to your doctor about steps you can take to prevent future episodes and, more importantly, a full-blown stroke.

As they age, many people worry about developing Alzheimer's disease, which affects memory and other higher brain functions. Older adults who feel they have difficulty with memory or suddenly display symptoms of dementia (a decline in mental abilities) may be experiencing reduced blood flow to the brain. This condition is known as multi-infarct dementia and, unlike Alzheimer's disease, can be stabilized with low-dose aspirin and careful management of blood pressure.

In cases of uncontrolled severe hypertension, the blood vessels can break down quickly in a process known as fibrinoid necrosis. This allows blood and fluid to leak into the brain, eventually raising the pressure within the skull cavity where the brain sits. Symptoms include headache and fatigue, and if the pressure is not relieved, the brain itself can be damaged. However, this outcome is extremely rare today because of major improvements in blood pressure control.

Finally, if it is dangerously elevated, high blood pressure can directly cause a disease of the brain known as hypertensive encephalopathy. Symptoms of this disease include severe hypertension, a disordered or confused mental state, increased intracranial (inside the skull) pressure, damage to the retina (see the next section), and seizures.

EYES

Although not involved in the regulation of blood pressure, your eyes have many arteries supplying them with blood. These arteries can be seen during an eye examination with a light shined on the retina, which is on the back of the eye. If the doctor observes areas where these blood vessels have burst or are narrowed, chances are likely that similar damage exists in other arteries in the body. Elevated blood pressure can cause the retina, which receives visual images from the lens, to degenerate in a condition known as retinopathy. These changes to arteries inside the eye are a strong indicator of similar changes occurring in the kidneys.

4

Diagnosing and Monitoring Blood Pressure

Because blood pressure fluctuates throughout the day and under certain circumstances, doctors never diagnose hypertension on the basis of a single reading. Usually, your doctor will measure your blood pressure on at least two or three separate visits to determine whether you have hypertension. The method used to measure blood pressure is also very important; proper equipment and technique are essential to get accurate blood pressure readings. You can take steps to ensure that your readings are accurate by cooperating with your doctor to monitor your blood pressure.

HOW BLOOD PRESSURE IS MEASURED

Blood pressure was first discovered in the 1600s when a scientist inserted a glass tube directly into the artery of a horse. Fortunately, a much less threatening method of measuring blood pressure has since been developed.

A cuff attached to a meter known as a sphygmomanometer (sfig-moe-meh-**nom**-ih-ter) is wrapped securely around your upper arm. Your doctor then inflates the cuff by squeezing the attached rubber bulb. This temporarily stops the flow of blood in the main artery in your arm (the brachial artery).

Then the air is slowly released from the cuff as your doctor listens through a stethoscope placed inside your elbow (directly over the artery). A beating sound can be heard as blood flows through the artery.

The doctor takes a reading from the meter as soon as he or she hears the first beating sound; this is the systolic blood pressure, or the first number of the two. The systolic blood pressure reading measures the highest pressure in the arteries. It is produced when the heart beats, pumping blood into your arteries. The reading is recorded as millimeters of mercury and is abbreviated as mm Hg.

As more air is gradually released from the cuff, the artery opens fully, restoring blood flow through the blood vessel. The beating sound gradually disappears. The doctor takes another reading from the meter when the last beating sound is heard; this is the diastolic blood pressure. The diastolic blood pressure reading measures the lowest pressure in the arteries. It occurs between heartbeats. The diastolic pressure is the second number of two. For example, if your blood pressure reading is 140 over 90 (written as 140/90 mm Hg), 140 is the systolic pressure, and 90 is the diastolic pressure.

TIPS TO HELP ENSURE ACCURATE BLOOD PRESSURE READINGS

One of the most overlooked causes of inaccurate blood pressure readings is the size of the cuff. Using a cuff that does not fit the person's arm can result in inaccurate readings. The cuff should be wide enough to reach from just below the armpit to the inside of the elbow. The cuff should completely encircle your arm with several inches to spare. When purchasing a home blood pressure kit, be sure it includes a cuff that will fit your arm. The table below will help you select the best size cuff for you from among the standard sizes available.

STANDARD CUFF SIZES

DISTANCE FROM SHOULDER TO ELBOW	CUFF SIZE
Less than 13 inches	5 by 9 inches (small)
13 to 16 inches	6 by 13 inches (medium)
More than 16 inches	7 by 14 inches (large)

You may want to consider the clothes you wear when you have your blood pressure checked. A short-sleeved shirt or sleeves that can easily be pushed up are best. A sleeve that must be rolled up until it tightens around your arm may affect your blood pressure reading.

Usually, it does not matter whether you are standing, sitting, or lying down when your blood pressure is measured. Older adults, people with diabetes, or people who are taking certain drugs (such as antihypertensive drugs and drugs used to treat Parkinson's disease) may have lower blood pressure when standing up. This is called postural hypotension. Often, doctors measure blood pressure in various body positions to determine whether this is a factor. However, blood pressure is usually measured with the person sitting quietly.

Blood pressure may be higher in the morning than in the afternoon or evening. Talking can elevate blood pressure, as can stress just before the measurement is taken. If you rush in late for an appointment, chances are your blood pressure will be slightly elevated if it is measured right away.

Smoking and drinking beverages that contain caffeine (coffee, tea, and colas) can affect blood pressure for two or more hours. Eating a lot of salt does not alter blood pressure in the short term, such as for an office visit, but may affect it over time (see Chapter 6). Older people may experience a drop in blood pressure right after eating.

Your doctor can show you how to monitor your own blood pressure. With practice, you should easily master the technique. For some useful tips, see pages 68 through 70.

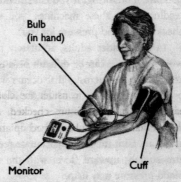

Bulb
(in hand)

Cuff

Monitor

Blood pressure taken at home may be slightly lower than that taken in the doctor's office. When checking your blood pressure at home, it is a good idea to take two or three readings, particularly when you first start monitoring your own blood pressure. Your doctor may ask you to check your blood pressure at different times of the day, such as morning and evening, to assess the effects of any medications you are taking. Frequent readings are recommended when you are first diagnosed, when you begin or make any changes in your treatment—especially drug treatment—and when you are undergoing treatment for another health problem. Under normal circumstances, when your pressure is well controlled, you will need to check it only every other week or once a month.

Electronic blood pressure monitors in supermarkets, drugstores, and other public places are convenient, but they are not a good substitute for checking your blood pressure with a sphygmomanometer. Because these machines are sensitive to any motion in the hand or arm, they are unlikely to measure blood pressure with a high degree of accuracy. However, these machines are useful in making the public aware of the importance of blood pressure monitoring. If you consistently get high blood pressure readings from these machines, you should have your doctor check your blood pressure for you.

In some older adults, accurately measuring blood pressure with any device can be difficult because of the hardening of the arteries (arteriosclerosis) that occurs with age. This can produce pseudohypertension, in which the blood pressure within the arteries cannot be measured accurately with standard blood pressure monitors. In anyone in whom the beating sounds in the artery are faint (making an accurate reading difficult), raising the arm straight upward (level with the shoulder) and taking the blood pressure may help.

CLASSIFICATION OF HYPERTENSION

Although there is no precise definition of high blood pressure, researchers over the years have determined the levels at which blood pressure becomes high enough to pose serious health risks. In the US, the Joint National Committee on Detection, Evaluation, and Treatment of High Blood Pressure releases guidelines for classifying people with hypertension. These guidelines are shown in the table below.

Because diastolic blood pressure represents the lower and more constant level of pressure in the arteries, doctors sometimes emphasize it more, especially in younger patients. Diastolic blood

BLOOD PRESSURE CLASSIFICATIONS FOR PEOPLE AGE 18 AND OLDER*

CATEGORY	SYSTOLIC	DIASTOLIC
Normal blood pressure	Lower than 130 mm Hg	Lower than 85 mm Hg
High-normal blood pressure	130 to 139 mm Hg	85 to 89 mm Hg
Hypertension:		
Stage 1 (mild)	140 to 159 mm Hg	90 to 99 mm Hg
Stage 2 (moderate)	160 to 179 mm Hg	100 to 109 mm Hg
Stage 3 (severe)	180 to 209 mm Hg	110 to 119 mm Hg
Stage 4 (very severe)	210 mm Hg or higher	120 mm Hg or higher

*A diagnosis of hypertension is based on two or more blood pressure readings taken at separate visits to the doctor's office. If your systolic blood pressure falls into one category and your diastolic pressure into another, the higher reading will be used to classify your blood pressure status. For example, a blood pressure reading of 160/92 mm Hg would be classified as stage 2 (moderate) hypertension, and a reading of 180/120 mm Hg would be classified as stage 4 (very severe) hypertension. For people who have isolated systolic hypertension, a reading of 170/85 mm Hg would be classified as stage 2 (moderate) hypertension.

pressure below 85 mm Hg is considered normal; measurements between 85 and 90 mm Hg are considered high-normal. When diastolic blood pressure ranges from 90 to 99 mm Hg, the person has mild hypertension. Diastolic blood pressure between 100 and 109 mm Hg is considered moderately elevated, and above 110 mm Hg is considered severely elevated. If diastolic blood pressure is more than 120 mm Hg, immediate emergency medical treatment may be required (see Chapter 11).

Elevated systolic blood pressure readings also indicate hypertension. Normal systolic pressure is no higher than 130 mm Hg. When systolic blood pressure reaches 130 to 139 mm Hg, it is considered high-normal. When systolic blood pressure ranges from 140 to 159 mm Hg, the person has mild hypertension; between 160 and 179 mm Hg, the person has moderate hypertension. Systolic pressure from 180 to 209 mm Hg is considered severely elevated, and above 210 mm Hg may be a medical emergency that requires immediate treatment.

If diastolic blood pressure falls under one category and systolic pressure under another, the *higher* category is used to classify blood pressure status. For example, if your blood pressure is 160 over 90, you have moderate hypertension. Similarly, if blood pressure readings are consistently higher in one arm than in the other, the higher reading is used.

Some people have normal diastolic blood pressure but elevated systolic blood pressure. This is more common in older adults. If systolic blood pressure is regularly over 140 mm Hg (and especially if it is over 160 mm Hg) while diastolic blood pressure remains below 90 mm Hg, the person has isolated systolic hypertension. Isolated systolic hypertension is staged the same way as essential hypertension.

While doctors once thought that high systolic blood pressure was not as dangerous as high diastolic blood pressure, new evidence suggests otherwise. In a study of 2,767 of the original participants in the Framingham Heart Study, men and women with borderline isolated systolic hypertension had about 1.5 times the risk of heart disease, death from heart disease, congestive heart failure, and stroke or transient ischemic attacks (TIAs; see Chapter 3) as people with normal blood pressure.

Some people, perhaps as many as one of five, may experience a slight rise in blood pressure when they have it checked at their doctor's office. This is known as white-coat hypertension. Because blood pressure can become elevated when you are feeling nervous or under stress, and because an office visit can cause such tension, many doctors ask their patients to monitor their own blood pressure at home to help ensure accurate readings (see Chapter 5). Doctors may also take two or three blood pressure readings during a single visit and then record the lowest reading.

A diagnosis of hypertension is made in adults when the average of two or more diastolic blood pressure readings on at least two subsequent office visits (after the initial screening) is higher than 90 mm Hg. A diagnosis of hypertension can also be made when the average of several systolic blood pressure readings on two or more subsequent office visits is consistently higher than 140 mm Hg. In cases in which blood pressure is severely elevated, or in which clear evidence of hypertension-related damage (such as changes in the blood vessels in the eyes or signs of an enlarged heart) exist, treatment may be started immediately.

For people whose blood pressure is only mildly elevated, a diagnosis of hypertension is generally based on three elevated measurements taken over a 6-month period. People who have mildly to moderately elevated blood pressure will be advised to make certain lifestyle changes before additional measurements are taken (see Chapter 6). These changes include cutting back on salt, losing weight, reducing alcohol intake, increasing physical activity, and limiting intake of coffee and other sources of caffeine. If the lifestyle changes help to lower your blood pressure, you will be asked to continue them, and your blood pressure will be monitored over a 2- to 3-month period. Most doctors will not start drug treatment unless lifestyle changes cannot control blood pressure over the course of several months.

People whose blood pressure fluctuates significantly are considered to have unstable hypertension. The same is said of people whose blood pressure readings often (but not always) fall within the hypertensive range. These people are treated as having borderline hypertension (high-normal to mild).

Your doctor may recommend that you wear a portable automatic blood pressure monitor to obtain readings throughout the day. These monitors are preset to measure your blood pressure at regular intervals without any effort on your part. You wear a blood pressure cuff around your arm all day, and the cuff automatically inflates and deflates at the scheduled times. The readings are stored in a radio control device worn around your waist. The stored information is downloaded into a computer, and the results printed out. These readings, taken throughout the day as you go about your usual activities, give your doctor the most accurate assessment of your blood pressure status. However, these devices are expensive, intrusive (they might interfere with work and sleep), and susceptible to technical problems. They are used mainly when hypertension does not seem to respond to treatment or when evidence of organ damage exists but blood pressure readings do not indicate severe hypertension.

EVALUATING A PERSON WITH HYPERTENSION

Once your high blood pressure has been diagnosed, your doctor will want to examine you more closely. He or she will want to determine the cause of your hypertension (see Chapter 2), whether high blood pressure has caused any damage (see Chapter 3), and whether you have any other risk factors that increase your chances of stroke or heart disease.

Interview

While hypertension usually does not cause any obvious symptoms, you may have had other health problems or concerns that brought you to your doctor in the first place. Noticeable symptoms of hypertension are generally related to severe elevations in blood pressure or to problems caused by hypertension that have gone untreated for some time.

Headaches in the lower back portion of the head—especially in the morning—are possible early symptoms associated with high blood pressure. However, headaches usually occur with severe hypertension rather than with more moderate hypertension. Other symptoms often include feeling dizzy, lightheaded, tired, or faint, or experiencing vision or hearing problems (a ringing or buzzing noise in the ears). Problems related to the effects of hypertension may include palpitations (an abnormally strong, rapid heartbeat), blood in the urine, leg pain while walking, impotence, angina (chest pain), shortness of breath, difficulty speaking, and weakness on one side of the body.

Your doctor will begin by asking whether hypertension runs

in your family or whether you have ever been told in the past that your blood pressure is high. He or she will also want to know what, if any, medications you take, including those you can buy without a prescription. He or she will ask about how much alcohol you drink, how many cigarettes you smoke, how much smokeless tobacco you use, and how much salt you eat. Your doctor will want to know whether you are physically active or sedentary. You should mention whether you have been under unusual stress recently or whether your lifestyle places you under frequent stress. Be sure also to tell your doctor if you have recently gained or lost weight. A change either way may provide clues as to the cause of your high blood pressure.

All of this information will help your doctor determine why your blood pressure is elevated and which treatment to prescribe. Your doctor will also discuss your complete health history and that of your family to decide which health problems to check for now and which ones to look for in the future. Your doctor will need to know about any health problems that can affect blood pressure, such as kidney problems, gout, diabetes, heart disease, high cholesterol levels, heart attack, or stroke.

Physical Examination

A physical examination will provide clues about the possible causes of your hypertension. The examination may start with a simple visual inspection. A round face with considerable abdominal fat and purple stretch marks on the skin may indicate excessive activity in the adrenal glands (especially a disorder known as Cushing's syndrome). An enlarged thyroid indicates thyroid problems. Swelling in the ankles or elsewhere on the body may indicate fluid retention. Your body weight may also be an important sign.

Your doctor will then begin to listen to your body for sounds that may be associated with problems that can cause high blood pressure. For example, in the abdomen, a high-pitched sound could suggest a narrowing of the renal artery (the artery that supplies blood to the kidney). Abnormal heart sounds can indicate an enlarged heart, abnormal heart rhythm, or a valve problem. Fluid in the lungs may be a sign of heart failure. And the quality of the sound of blood flow through the major arteries in the neck will indicate whether you are at risk for stroke. Your doctor will also feel with his or her fingers in the region of your kidneys to see if they are enlarged or if there are any unusual lumps.

Your doctor will shine a light onto the back of your eyes to check the condition of blood vessels there. Your eyes are the only organ in which the blood vessels can be seen directly without an invasive procedure. Your doctor will look for any twisted blood vessels, any signs of bleeding or narrowing, or any other damage. If there is damage to these blood vessels, there is probably damage to other blood vessels in the body.

Especially in younger people, measuring blood pressure and pulse rate both in the arm and in the leg (in the groin area) is important for determining whether there is coarctation of the aorta (blood pressure higher in the arm than in the leg). Coarctation of the aorta and other possible causes of hypertension are discussed in Chapter 2.

For older people, a neurologic examination is critical for helping the doctor determine whether a stroke has already occurred. In a neurologic examination, the doctor will ask questions, measure your strength and sensitivity (including sensitivity to pain) on both sides of your body, check your reflexes, and evaluate your senses (usually vision, hearing, and touch).

Laboratory Tests

In addition to your interview and physical examination, your doctor will want to perform a few routine laboratory tests. These tests will help diagnose treatable causes of hypertension, identify health problems caused by (or coexisting with) your high blood pressure, and suggest the best method of treatment.

Because the kidneys can both cause high blood pressure and be affected by it, a complete analysis of your urine (a urinalysis) is essential. Your urine will be checked for the presence of protein or glucose (sugar), which could suggest kidney disease or diabetes. Blood tests will also provide useful information about your kidneys; high levels of creatinine in the blood indicate kidney problems.

Your blood will also be checked for the amount of potassium and calcium, glucose, and cholesterol and triglycerides to help determine if you have secondary hypertension. The test results will also help your doctor monitor your response to treatment.

Your doctor may recommend an electrocardiogram (ECG) to determine whether your heart is enlarged or damaged. An ECG is a record of your heart's electrical activity. In certain cases, an echocardiogram may be recommended to evaluate the size of your heart and how well it functions.

Special Tests

Your doctor may make some discoveries during the physical examination and with the standard laboratory tests that lead him or her to recommend more specialized tests. These special tests are used mainly to confirm a suspected secondary cause of hypertension or to determine why the hypertension is not responding to treatment. Some of these tests are invasive (body tissues are penetrated); others are noninvasive (body tissues are not penetrated). Most are performed on an outpatient basis. As you might expect, many of these tests focus on the kidneys.

The simplest of these tests is a 24-hour urine sample, in which you collect all your urine for a 24-hour period. The specimens are sent to a laboratory for renin and sodium levels to be checked. Normally, low sodium levels result in high renin levels and vice versa. If the renin and sodium levels are not proportional, you may have renovascular hypertension (see Chapter 2). The laboratory will also measure the amounts of certain hormones, such as epinephrine and norepinephrine, and their by-products. If levels of these are too high, you may have pheochromocytoma (see Chapter 2).

Diagnostic imaging techniques may also be useful. For example, your doctor may recommend an ultrasound scan to examine the size and shape of your kidneys. In this procedure, sound waves are used to obtain pictures of your kidneys, which are recorded on video and X-ray film. Ultrasound scanning is safe and noninvasive.

For a more detailed view of your kidneys or other organs, your doctor will probably recommend either a CT (computed tomography) or an MRI (magnetic resonance imaging) scan. Both CT and MRI scanning are safe and noninvasive. Like a standard X-ray machine, a CT scanner uses radiation to take pictures, but the beam of radiation is very focused (so you do not need a lead apron to cover the rest of your body). A computer helps process the images, which are recorded on X-ray film.

An MRI scanner uses radiowaves (like those that transmit radio signals), a powerful magnet, and a computer to process the information obtained. The pictures are recorded on X-ray film. MRI is particularly useful for finding tiny tumors in the pituitary gland.

Sometimes, invasive tests may be needed to determine how well your kidneys are functioning. An intravenous pyelogram (IVP), or urogram, involves injecting contrast material (dye) into your veins and then taking X rays as your kidneys filter out and excrete the dye. A retrograde pyelogram, in which contrast material is introduced through the ureter (one of the two tubes that carries urine from the kidneys to the bladder), may need to be performed in the operating room under anesthesia.

A renogram (renal scan) involves the use of a radioactive tracer that reveals both the appearance and function of the kidneys. In some cases, the doctor may take pictures and test your renin levels right before and 1 hour after you take an angiotensin converting enzyme (ACE) inhibitor. If you have renovascular hypertension, the affected kidney does not filter out and excrete the radioisotope as quickly as normal, and your renin level rises much higher than in essential hypertension.

Another test of kidney function is a renal vein renin test. Blood samples are taken directly from each renal vein (the veins that move blood from the kidneys toward the heart), and the amount of renin in each sample is compared. If blood flow to one kidney is obstructed, that kidney will produce excessive amounts of renin, while the other kidney will almost stop all renin production to compensate.

A renal arteriogram is an invasive procedure in which dye is injected directly into the renal arteries (the arteries that supply blood to the kidneys) through a catheter (tube) threaded through the large artery in your leg (femoral artery), and X rays are taken. A renal arteriogram shows very clearly where and to what degree one or both renal arteries are blocked. With a digital subtraction angiogram, the contrast material is injected through a catheter placed in a vein in the arm (and sometimes threaded through as far as the vena cava, the large vein that drains blood into the heart). A series of pictures is taken of the renal arteries with a computerized device that can then process the information to show narrowed or blocked blood vessels.

Complicated, Accelerated, and Malignant Hypertension

Once your doctor has completed the evaluation of your blood pressure and health status, he or she may modify your diagnosis to take other factors into account. Complications of hypertension refers to organ damage caused by high blood pressure (such as chronic heart failure, renal failure, arterial aneurysm, or history of heart attack or stroke).

Two final types of hypertension are medical emergencies that require immediate treatment. Accelerated hypertension refers to significantly elevated blood pressure associated with visible damage to the blood vessels in the eye. If left untreated, accelerated hypertension progresses to a malignant (life-threatening) phase. Malignant hypertension is associated with widespread damage to blood vessel walls; this condition requires immediate hospitalization and medical care. Both accelerated and malignant hypertension are characterized by extremely high blood pressure levels that occur suddenly (determined according to a person's usual blood pressure levels). Often, people with these two types of hypertension have no obvious symptoms. However, some people may experience headache, chest pain, or shortness of breath, all of which are related to organ damage caused by high blood pressure. Malignant hypertension is usually fatal unless treated promptly and aggressively; outlook after treatment depends on kidney, brain, and heart function.

DIAGNOSIS OF SECONDARY HYPERTENSION*

POSSIBLE CAUSES OF SECONDARY HYPERTENSION	TESTS	REASONS FOR TESTS
RENAL (KIDNEY) DISORDERS		
Renovascular hypertension (due to atherosclerosis or fibrous hyperplasia)	Rapid-sequence intravenous pyelogram (IVP)	Check and compare kidney function and size
	Digital subtraction angiogram	Examine renal arteries for blockage
	Captopril renogram	Check and compare kidney function
	Renal vein renin test	Check and compare renin levels (elevated in kidney with renal artery blockage)
	Renal ultrasound	Examine and compare kidney size (diseased kidneys will be either too large or too small)
	Blood lipid profile	Check cholesterol levels (elevated total cholesterol, elevated low density lipoprotein [LDL, or

POSSIBLE CAUSES OF SECONDARY HYPERTENSION	TESTS	REASONS FOR TESTS
		"bad"] cholesterol, elevated triglyceride levels and low levels of high density [HDL, or "good"] cholesterol indicate risk of atherosclerosis)
Glomerulonephritis	Urinalysis	Check for color (dark brown), red blood cells (elevated levels), protein (high levels), and other blood cells (elevated levels)
	Antibody levels	Check for infectious agent in acute glomerulonephritis
	Renal ultrasound	Check kidney size (normal or enlarged in acute disease, small in chronic disease)
Polycystic kidney disease	Urinalysis	Check for pus and red blood cells
	Intravenous urogram (IVU)	Check for enlarged kidneys with irregular outlines (due to cysts)
	Renal ultrasound, abdominal computed tomography (CT) scan	Check for enlarged, abnormal-looking kidneys (both ultrasound and CT scan)
Hydronephrosis	Abdominal ultrasound	Check for enlarged kidney
	IVU	Examine kidneys and lower urinary tract

POSSIBLE CAUSES OF SECONDARY HYPERTENSION	TESTS	REASONS FOR TESTS
	Cystourethrogram	Check for blockage of urethra
	Retrograde ureteropyelogram	Examine kidneys and lower urinary tract

ENDOCRINE (GLANDULAR) DISORDERS

Aldosteronism	Blood aldosterone level	Check for excess aldosterone
	Blood potassium level	Check for low potassium
	Blood renin activity	Check for renin levels in lying and sitting positions
	24-hour urine collection	Check for low amount of sodium
	Abdominal CT scan	Check for tumor(s) in adrenal gland(s)
Pheochromocytoma	24-hour urine collection	Check for elevated catecholamine (a chemical that carries messages from the brain or nerve cells to other nerve cells) levels in urine
	Digital subtraction angiogram	Used to locate tumor(s)
Cushing's syndrome	Blood cortisol level	Checked throughout the day; cortisol levels remain elevated with Cushing's syndrome
	24-hour urine collection	Check for elevated cortisol level

POSSIBLE CAUSES OF SECONDARY HYPERTENSION	TESTS	REASONS FOR TESTS
	Dexamethasone given at bedtime; blood cortisol level measured the next morning	Check to see if drug suppressed cortisol levels
	Brain magnetic resonance imaging (MRI) scan	Check for tumor in pituitary gland
	Abdominal CT scan	Check for tumor in adrenal gland
Congenital adrenal hyperplasia	Urinalysis	Check for abnormal androgen and corticosteroid levels
	Blood testosterone level	Check for elevated level
Hypothyroidism (myxedema)	Blood thyroid-stimulating hormone (TSH) level	Check for elevated level (primary hypothyroidism) versus low/normal level (secondary hypothyroidism)
	Thyroid-releasing hormone (TRH) test	Check TSH before and after injection of TRH; TSH is not released if the pituitary gland is diseased
Hyperthyroidism	Blood thyroid hormone levels	Check for elevated thyroid activity
Acromegaly	Skull and hand X rays	Check for enlargement and other characteristic changes in bone

POSSIBLE CAUSES OF SECONDARY HYPERTENSION	TESTS	REASONS FOR TESTS
	Blood growth hormone level	Check for elevated level
	Blood phosphate level	Check for elevated level
	Blood insulinlike growth factor (IGF) level	Check for elevated level
Hyperparathyroidism	Blood calcium level	Check for elevated level
	Blood parathyroid hormone level	Check for elevated level
	Blood phosphate level	Check for low (primary hyperparathyroidism) versus elevated (secondary hyperparathyroidism) level
Hypercalcemia	Blood calcium level	Check for elevated level

VASCULAR (HEART AND BLOOD VESSEL) DISORDERS

Coarctation of the aorta	Chest X ray	Check for coarctation
Aortic regurgitation	Echocardiogram	Examine heart and valve function

NEUROLOGIC (BRAIN AND NERVOUS SYSTEM) DISORDERS

Guillain-Barré syndrome	Cerebrospinal fluid	Check for increased protein levels without increased number of cells
Intracranial pressure	Intracranial pressure test	Check for elevated pressure

*Many of the secondary causes of hypertension discussed in Chapter 2 require special diagnostic tests. Most of these tests are described here, in Chapter 4. This table may help you to better understand why your doctor may have recommended that you undergo certain medical tests. Be sure to talk to your doctor if you have any questions or concerns about the tests you are having.

5

♦

Treatment Planning

To successfully manage your blood pressure, you need to work closely with your doctor to develop a treatment plan. Your treatment plan will probably include lifestyle changes, antihypertensive medication, and regular blood pressure checks.

WORKING WITH YOUR DOCTOR

While this may seem obvious, whether you follow your doctor's instructions often hinges on the cost of treatment and how well you tolerate it. Patients may be reluctant to discuss the expense of treatment with their doctors. Be sure to talk to your doctor about your financial and insurance situation. He or she may be able to adjust the treatment plan to fit your budget better.

You should also be prepared to discuss any side effects or inconveniences caused by medications or lifestyle changes. Keep track of any symptoms related either to your high blood pressure or its treatment. Your doctor may not be able to help relieve every unpleasant aspect of treatment, but he or she can offer support and advice and can probably adjust your therapy to make it more compatible with your daily routine.

You can take an active role in your treatment by keeping all appointments with your doctor, by taking all medications as directed, and by following advice about diet and exercise. You should set a target goal for your blood pressure with your physician: he or she will know what level is best for your health, and you can give input on what level of therapy you can manage. Before you leave your doctor's office, always make sure that both of you have a clear understanding about what you need to do between now and your next visit (for example, lifestyle changes, medication use, and blood pressure monitoring). By working closely with your doctor, you can control your blood pressure.

Measuring your own blood pressure at home will probably be an important part of your treatment. Many mechanical and electronic blood pressure monitors are sold for home use, and they vary in accuracy and price. Before you purchase a home blood pressure kit, it is a good idea to ask your doctor which type would be best for you. For unbiased ratings of various home blood pressure monitors, check back issues of *Consumer Reports* magazine at your local public library.

A typical blood pressure kit usually includes a blood pressure meter, cuffs (in different sizes), a stethoscope, and step-by-step instructions. Some electronic blood pressure monitors have self-inflating cuffs and do not require that you use a stethoscope. Your doctor or another health-care professional (such as a nurse) can show you the proper technique for checking your own blood pressure. With practice, you should easily master the procedure.

Here are some useful tips for monitoring your own blood pressure:

- Be sure to carefully follow the instructions supplied with your blood pressure kit.
- Check your blood pressure at the same time(s) every day.
- Avoid caffeine and nicotine (for example, coffee, tea, colas, cigarettes, and nicotine gum) within a half hour before checking your blood pressure; these stimulants could cause an inaccurate reading.
- Rest for several minutes before you begin; take a few deep breaths and relax.
- Place your arm on a sturdy surface (such as the armrest of a chair), level with your heart.
- Press your fingertips firmly but gently inside your elbow to locate the pulse in the main artery in your arm. You may need to make several attempts before finding your pulse.
- Wrap the cuff securely around your upper arm, just above your elbow. To ensure an accurate reading, use a cuff that fits. The cuff should wrap once around your arm with several inches to spare.
- Make sure that the blood pressure meter is set at zero.
- Put the stethoscope directly onto the area where you found the pulse in your arm. (Do not forget to put the earpieces into your ears.)

- Watch the meter as you inflate the cuff to at least 30 mm Hg above your last systolic blood pressure reading. (You should not hear anything through the stethoscope at this time.)
- Then, listen carefully and continue to watch the meter as you turn the release valve and slowly deflate the cuff (at a rate of not more than 2 mm Hg per second). When you first hear a beating sound, record the number on the meter. This is your systolic blood pressure.
- Continue to slowly deflate the cuff while listening and watching the meter. When the beating sound fades noticeably or disappears completely, record the number on the meter. This is your diastolic blood pressure.
- Take two or more readings to ensure accuracy.
- Keep a careful record of your blood pressure readings to share with your doctor during your next office visit. For each reading, be sure to include the following helpful information: time of day checked, arm checked (left or right), body position (sitting, standing, or lying down), physical and mental state (for example, under stress, after exercise, or not feeling well), and timing in relation to medication use (how soon after taking medication and type of medication taken).

AVAILABLE OPTIONS

The main goal of treatment is to keep you healthy and to reduce your risk of cardiovascular disease, including stroke, or death. The decision to begin treatment is based on your blood pressure readings, the presence of other health problems, and your likelihood of developing cardiovascular disease. The initial blood pressure level you achieve through treatment may not be considered "normal" by the official classification guidelines (see page 51), but you should continue to aim for your lowest possible blood pressure. Your doctor will discuss with you what blood pressure level you should expect to reach.

Your doctor will probably first recommend some lifestyle changes, which are explained in detail in Chapter 6. If you can make permanent healthful changes to your daily routine, you may not need to take medication, or you may be able to manage your blood pressure with a lower dose. Many of these lifestyle changes will also reduce your risk of heart disease beyond the beneficial effect of lowering your blood pressure.

Proof of the effectiveness of lifestyle changes as a treatment regimen has been published in the medical literature. The Treatment of Mild Hypertension Study showed that motivated people with stage 1 or 2 hypertension were able to make and maintain several lifestyle changes. These changes resulted in significant weight loss, reduced sodium and alcohol intake, and increased physical activity. They were associated with a significant decrease in blood pressure that lasted more than 4 years. Another study, the Trials of Hypertension Prevention, also found that weight loss was the most effective method for reducing blood pressure in people with high-normal levels. Eating less sodium also proved effective. Researchers estimate that weight loss, regular exercise, and a low-salt diet could reduce the number of Americans with high blood pressure by 20 percent to 50 percent.

The risk of developing cardiovascular problems is closely related to the degree that your blood pressure is elevated. Therefore, drug therapy is necessary when lifestyle changes are not effective in lowering blood pressure. Clinical trials show that drug therapy in stage 2 through stage 4 hypertension reduces overall cardiovascular disease and death, significantly reducing the risk of stroke, heart attack, congestive heart failure, and end-stage kidney disease.

Best of all, the growing number of antihypertensive drugs makes it possible to customize treatment for each person. Research has shown that most medications used alone effectively control blood pressure in more than half of people with stage 1 or 2 hypertension. Two major studies found no significant advantage for choosing one drug over another. Some of your test results may suggest that one drug will work better for you (see Chapter 7), and some drugs have fewer side effects—though these are usually more expensive. If you need to take medication, and if the first drug your doctor prescribes does not control your blood pressure (or if it causes unpleasant side effects), your doctor may either switch your medication or add a second drug to your treatment regimen.

COMPLEMENTARY THERAPIES

Some alternative or complementary therapies may help you feel better and more relaxed, but they will not necessarily lower your blood pressure. For example, relaxation techniques and biofeedback have been studied formally and have not been found to improve blood pressure. Other treatments, such as acupuncture, are still under investigation.

Relaxation Techniques

The relaxation response is the opposite of the fight-or-flight response (see Chapter 1). It involves lowering your heart rate, blood pressure, and oxygen consumption by sitting quietly in a comfortable position, relaxing your muscles, and repeating a word (such as *one* or *peace*) with each breath. Advocates of relaxation techniques recommend practicing the relaxation response twice a day for 10 to 20 minutes. This process is similar to the practice of yoga, Zen, and transcendental meditation, in which a single word is repeated to block out thoughts of worldly things. Studies of the effectiveness of relaxation training and methods to reduce anger and mood swings have not shown much benefit. Diastolic blood pressure may drop slightly, but usually systolic blood pressure is not affected.

Biofeedback

Another alternative approach uses biofeedback to lower blood pressure. Your nervous system includes both voluntary (under conscious control, such as movement of skeletal muscles) and involuntary (not under conscious control, such as heart rate, respiration, digestion, and blood pressure) functions. The goal of biofeedback is to make you aware of these involuntary functions so you can consciously control them. For this technique, you are connected to a special monitor that tracks involuntary body functions such as blood pressure, heart rate, and skin temperature, and feeds the information back to you. Then, you can use this information to learn to gain control over these functions. Scientific research has shown that biofeedback can be helpful in treating certain health problems, such as headache and stroke.

Acupuncture

Although acupuncture is one of the oldest forms of medical treatment in the world, scientists are still examining whether it has any direct impact on the body beyond a possible placebo effect (a response to treatment caused by a person's expectations, rather than by the treatment itself). According to the Chinese concept of disease, good health is regarded as a balance between the opposing forces of yin and yang, and the attraction between them creates an energy or life force known as *chi*. This life force flows through the body in 14 major meridians or channels. Acupuncture aims to restore the balance in your *chi* through the insertion of needles at any of over 300 locations along these channels. The effect of acupuncture on hypertension has not yet been formally studied.

6

Steps You Can Take

Many people can successfully lower their blood pressure through lifestyle changes, eliminating the need to take blood pressure medication. Other people will need to combine a healthy lifestyle with medication use. The recommendations in this chapter will help you keep your blood pressure under control.

LOSE WEIGHT

Being overweight is associated with many health problems, including heart disease, cancer, diabetes, gallbladder disease, arthritis, and sleep apnea (when you stop breathing in your sleep). A clear, direct relationship exists between body weight and blood pressure. That is, higher body weight usually means higher blood pressure. Study results suggest that 6 of every 10 adults with hypertension weigh 20 percent more than their ideal body weight. In younger adults, the effect of weight on blood pressure is even greater. Between ages 20 and 44, the risk of hypertension is five times higher for overweight people than for people of normal weight; the risk is only twice as high for overweight people over age 45.

Weight loss lowers blood pressure to a similar degree. Even the loss of 10 pounds in an overweight person usually results in a noticeable drop in blood pressure. In the Trials of Hypertension Prevention, a 10-pound weight loss was associated with a decrease in systolic blood pressure of 3.8 mm Hg and in diastolic blood pressure of 2.8 mm Hg. This may not sound like much, but it could be enough to help you avoid taking medication.

In the Dietary Intervention Study in Hypertension, 60 percent of hypertensive people who lost weight could maintain control of their blood pressure without medication. Another study noted that the effects of left ventricular hypertrophy (see Chapter 3) in young, overweight people with hypertension were decreased more with an 18-pound weight loss than with antihypertensive medication. Evidence suggests that additional weight loss will lower blood pressure even further: one study found that a loss of 20 to 22 pounds resulted in a 26-mm Hg reduction in systolic blood pressure and a 20-mm Hg reduction in diastolic blood pressure.

Losing weight has also been shown to lower the cost of treatment, especially for people who have both hypertension and diabetes (see Chapter 14). This occurs because people who lose weight typically need to take less medication. In one study, people with these diseases were placed on a weight-loss diet for 12

FIND YOUR HEALTHY WEIGHT

Compare your actual weight to the recommended healthy weight range for your height and frame size (most people have a medium frame).

Note: Heights shown are in feet and inches, without shoes; weights shown are in pounds, without clothes.

	MEN				WOMEN		
	WEIGHT				WEIGHT		
HEIGHT	SMALL FRAME	MEDIUM FRAME	LARGE FRAME	HEIGHT	SMALL FRAME	MEDIUM FRAME	LARGE FRAME
5'4"	114–122	120–132	128–145	5'	98–106	103–115	111–127
5'5"	117–126	123–136	131–149	5'1"	101–109	106–118	114–130
5'6"	121–130	127–140	135–154	5'2"	104–112	109–122	117–134
5'7"	125–134	131–145	140–159	5'3"	107–115	112–126	121–138
5'8"	129–138	135–149	144–163	5'4"	110–119	116–131	125–142
5'9"	133–143	139–153	148–167	5'5"	114–123	120–135	129–146
5'10"	137–147	143–158	152–172	5'6"	118–127	124–139	133–150
5'11"	141–151	147–163	157–177	5'7"	122–131	128–143	137–154
6'	145–155	151–168	161–182	5'8"	126–136	132–147	141–159
6'1"	149–160	155–173	166–187	5'9"	130–140	136–151	145–164
6'2"	153–164	160–178	171–192	5'10"	134–144	140–155	149–169

If you have any questions or concerns about your ideal weight, talk to your doctor.

weeks. The average monthly cost for antihypertensive and antidiabetes medications and supplies was $63.30 per person before weight loss. Following completion of the diet, this cost per month dropped to $20.40. One year later, the average monthly cost was $32.40. The estimated average savings in prescription costs over the year was $442.80.

However, if you need to lose weight, you do not need to

achieve an "ideal" body weight to improve your blood pressure and overall health. Rather than feeling defeated at the thought of trying to lose 50 pounds, concentrate on taking off 5 or 10 pounds instead, at least initially. The benefits of even minimal weight loss have been observed in blacks and whites, men and women.

Of course, as anyone who has ever fought the battle of the bulge knows, losing weight is much easier than maintaining weight loss. However, motivated people determined to control their blood pressure have shown that it can be done. In the Trials of Hypertension Prevention, men kept off an average of more than 10 pounds for 18 months. They also enjoyed a 2.8-mm Hg drop in diastolic blood pressure and a 3.1-mm Hg drop in systolic blood pressure. Women kept off nearly 4 pounds, for a 1.1-mm Hg reduction in diastolic blood pressure and a 2.0-mm Hg reduction in systolic pressure. These people had high-normal blood pressure, so these small improvements in blood pressure were quite important. Researchers believe that high-normal blood pressure is very likely to progress to more severe hypertension, so even a small decrease in blood pressure is a good sign. In addition, weight reduction brings favorable changes in the amount of lipids (fats and fatlike substances), uric acid (a waste product of the breakdown of protein in the cells), and glucose (sugar) in the blood.

In the Trial of Antihypertensive Interventions and Management, the beneficial effects of weight loss on blood pressure lasted longer than the numbers on the scale would suggest. Although participants regained much of their original weight over a 5-year period, the beneficial effects of weight loss on blood pressure remained: 33 percent of these people maintained blood pressure control without medication, and weight loss reduced the likelihood of needing additional medications by 12 percent to 32 percent for those already taking medication. Researchers believe that the good effects of weight loss take hold faster than the bad effects of weight gain. Of course, this is no excuse to lose and regain weight repeatedly. Additional evidence suggests that this pattern of repeated weight loss and weight gain over the years can lead to possible heart disease and premature death.

If you need to lose weight, be sure to take a sensible approach. You did not gain weight in 2 weeks, so do not expect to lose it that quickly. Slow, gradual weight loss has proved to be the best strategy. A realistic goal and time frame is to lose 10 percent of your body weight over the course of a year; 1 or 2 pounds per week is enough. Again, losing weight may seem like the easy part—your real goal is to keep the weight off.

To put this into perspective, consider this: eating just 50 extra calories per day (the amount in a slice of diet bread) would add up to 26 pounds of gained weight over the course of 5 years. This is how most people become overweight—gradually. This is also how most people should plan to lose weight.

The key to long-term weight maintenance is to develop healthy eating and exercise habits that you can stick with for the rest of your life. Tips for both are discussed in detail later in this chapter. You should not think of it as "going on" or "going off" a diet. Rather, think of it as a healthy lifestyle. And your motto should be Moderation rather than Deprivation.

Just as you monitor your blood pressure levels, you should keep track of your weight, general eating patterns, and activity levels. If you notice that you are slipping, make every effort to get back on track. By setting practical goals, you are less likely to fall into the "all or nothing" thinking that derails so many unsuccessful dieters. ("I ate too much last night at the party, so it does not matter what I eat today.")

Developing problem-solving skills is also critical. If your job requires that you dine out often, learn how to order healthy, low-fat meals from a restaurant menu. If you are constantly traveling, make it a priority to figure out how to work in some exercise or less formal physical activity. If you have children, you will probably find it easier in terms of shopping, cooking, and scheduling to make your healthy lifestyle a family affair.

You may be tempted to "go it alone" and surprise everyone with your weight loss, but you will be more likely to succeed if you develop a support network. Be sure to tell your doctor about your progress—you have every right to be proud of even the smallest weight loss—and to ask for suggestions. Other health professionals, such as dietitians and nutritionists, can also be very helpful and supportive. Some people benefit from group support, while others prefer to set their own schedules and personal goals.

Whatever steps you take to lose weight, be sure to discuss them with your doctor. But in the end, it is all up to you.

BECOME MORE ACTIVE

Not surprisingly, physically active people are much less likely to have high blood pressure than are sedentary "couch potatoes." Regular exercise reduces blood pressure modestly in people with mild to moderate hypertension and is more likely to prevent additional increases in blood pressure. Some studies show that the effect of exercise on blood pressure is somewhat greater in women

HOW TO LOSE WEIGHT

Here are some useful tips to help you lose weight:

- Take weight off gradually; 1 to 2 pounds per week is adequate.
- Plan your meals in advance.
- Do not shop for food when you are hungry.
- Do not buy on impulse; make a shopping list and buy only what is on the list.
- Choose low-fat or nonfat foods.
- Eat plenty of fresh fruits and vegetables and whole-grain foods.
- Avoid eating fried foods; bake, broil, microwave, roast, or steam your food.
- Avoid eating junk foods; snack on fresh fruit instead.
- Do not skip meals.
- Try to eat only when you are hungry.
- At fast-food restaurants, choose dishes with less fat—salads, soups, baked potatoes, or grilled chicken sandwiches.
- Do not get discouraged if you occasionally cheat on your diet; simply resume your healthy eating habits at the next meal.
- Exercise regularly.

than in men. Exercise also reduces the risk of cardiovascular disease independent of weight loss and has proved highly beneficial for people with end-stage kidney disease.

You may be able to lower your blood pressure by about 10 mm Hg with endurance or aerobic training. Your blood pressure will not get any worse, and you will feel better afterward for having gotten your heart rate up and worked your muscles. Although strength training offers benefits, reducing blood pressure may not be one of them. Because your blood pressure shoots up when you raise or lower weights or use resistance machines, you should talk to your doctor before starting any strength training regimen.

Aerobic exercise, such as brisk walking, cycling, and swimming, helps lower blood pressure by strengthening your heart and allowing it to work more efficiently. Your heart does not need to beat as fast; this reduces cardiac output and thus blood pressure (Chapter 1). During aerobic exercise, your blood vessels expand to allow more blood to flow through to your muscles. During aerobic exercise, total peripheral resistance drops by nearly 85 percent, and resistance within the skeletal muscle blood vessels may decrease by as much as 95 percent.

Regular aerobic exercise will lead to structural changes in your blood vessels as well. Your body will add more arterioles and capillaries to accommodate the higher blood flow needed during exercise. These additional blood vessels help reduce total peripheral resistance. At the same time, the channel opening of your coronary arteries will become larger. This ensures that your heart will get enough blood during exercise without putting too much strain on these important arteries.

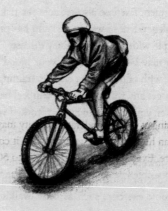

Regular aerobic exercise, such as bicycling, will help you control your blood pressure. Try to exercise for at least 30 minutes every day.

AEROBIC EXERCISE

Here are some good examples of aerobic exercise. Choose the ones that you enjoy and add them to your personal exercise program.

- Brisk walking
- Hiking
- Jogging
- Bicycling
- Stationary bicycling
- Swimming
- Stair climbing

- Rowing
- Jumping rope
- Cross-country skiing
- Aerobic dancing (in a class or to a video)
- Step aerobics (in a class or to a video)

You can exercise outdoors, at home, at a gym or health club, or at a local mall.

Immediately after exercise, blood pressure falls below its usual level. Blood pressure is lowest about 30 minutes after you have stopped exercising. Your vessels are still wide open, but your body no longer has the extra demands of exercise. Systolic blood pressure may drop by as much as 20 mm Hg, and it will remain lower than usual for at least 90 minutes after you have stopped exercising. Your blood pressure gradually climbs to its preexercise level over the next 3 to 4 hours, but the benefits continue to add up over time.

To achieve all these good effects, you do not need to train at the level of an Olympic athlete. Some research suggests that exercising at low to moderate intensity may be as (or more) effective than high-intensity training when it comes to lowering blood pressure. Exercising at just 40 percent to 60 percent of your maximum possible level of exertion should be beneficial and comfortable.

The key in exercising, as in losing weight, is to develop habits that you will enjoy and continue for the rest of your life. Most of the healthy benefits described above come with longer sessions of activity, of at least 20 to 30 minutes. Longer exercise periods are even better. However, short periods of activity, such as a brisk walk during your lunch break or taking the stairs throughout the day, add up and contribute to your total health.

The American College of Sports Medicine recommends that Americans engage in moderate exercise for at least 30 minutes every day. Your heart will benefit even if your exercise is spread out in short segments (10 to 20 minutes) throughout the day. Experts do not insist, though, that you go to a health club and sweat it out. Yard work, household chores, recreational dancing, hiking, and other activities that you might not think of as exercise all contribute to your total activity level. Try to fit some brisk walking into your day, every day—walk to the store, walk to the mailbox, and use the stairs instead of the elevator. If you are physically challenged, you can often find an activity, such as swimming or water exercise, that will get your heart pumping.

Less than one quarter of all Americans exercise at levels recommended for cardiovascular health. Lack of time, schedule conflicts, lack of family support, inconvenience, and failure to reach goals are the most common reasons given for not being more physically active. Rather than falling into the "all or nothing" trap, keep your daily activity plan flexible. Be prepared to settle for a few short, brisk walks scattered throughout the day if something comes up that prevents you from a planned exercise session or other physical activity. If you have not exercised for some time, and if you have heart disease or other cardiovascular conditions, talk to your doctor before you begin an exercise program.

WARMING UP AND COOLING DOWN

Always warm up before exercising by stretching all of your muscles (arms, legs, chest, shoulders, abdomen). Stretching will improve flexibility, help increase blood flow, and help prevent injury. Begin gradually, stretching slowly and carefully. Do not bounce or jerk and be careful not to overstretch. When you exercise, start slowly and gradually work up to a comfortable pace.

Cooling down after exercise helps prevent muscle soreness and decreases your chances of injury. Be sure to stop exercising slowly and gradually. For example, after jogging, gradually slow down until you are walking, and continue walking for several minutes. Or, toward the end of a brisk walk, gradually slow your pace. After cooling down, massage your muscles to help your blood circulate.

WHEN TO STOP EXERCISING

Warning: Never ignore the symptoms of possible overexercise, which could mean that you are having a heart attack or some other medical emergency. Stop exercising **immediately** if you have any of these symptoms:

- Pain or pressure in your chest
- Pain in your neck, jaw, or down your left arm
- Palpitations (a disturbing feeling that your heart is beating irregularly, more strongly, or more rapidly than normal)
- Nausea
- Blurred vision
- Severe shortness of breath
- Feeling faint or fainting

If you think you may be having a heart attack, call immediately for emergency medical assistance or have someone take you to the nearest hospital emergency department.

If you injure yourself, stop exercising immediately. Trying to "work through" the pain could cause more damage to injured tissues. If you have a strain, sprain, or muscle pull, rest the injury for a few days and follow the RICE (rest, ice, compression, and elevation) routine (see page 86). If you think the injury might be serious, talk to your doctor as soon as possible. If you think you have broken a bone, go to your hospital's emergency department.

RICE ROUTINE FOR FIRST AID

Rest, ice, compression, and elevation, or RICE, are the recommended steps for immediate treatment of such minor injuries as sprains, strains, and muscle pulls. If you think your injury might be serious, call your doctor before using RICE.

- **Rest.** Stop exercising and rest the injured part of your body to help reduce swelling and stop further bleeding in the tissues.
- **Ice.** Apply an ice pack to the injured area at regular intervals (about 20 to 30 minutes a session, every 3 hours) over the first several days after an injury. The cold temperature of the ice pack relieves pain and helps limit swelling and bruising by narrowing your blood vessels.
- **Compression.** Place an elastic compression bandage around the injured body part; wear the bandage for at least 2 days. Cover the injured area with the bandage, but also extend the bandage a few inches above and below the injury. Do not wrap the bandage too tightly, because it can cut off circulation in the injured part. Loosen the bandage if swelling increases. Like ice, compression helps limit swelling and bruising and relieves pain by supporting injured muscles and tendons. **Warning:** If you have diabetes or vascular disease, talk to your doctor before using an elastic bandage; an elastic bandage can interfere with circulation if you wrap it too tightly.
- **Elevation.** When you can, keep the injured part elevated above the level of your heart. Elevation reduces pressure in the tissues, which in turn helps drain any fluids that have collected in the tissues after your injury. Also, elevation reduces swelling and bruising.

MODIFY YOUR DIET

Nutrition Primer

Your body needs about 40 different nutrients to work properly. These nutrients include oxygen, protein, carbohydrate, fat, vitamins, and minerals. The three main energy sources—protein, carbohydrate, and fat—are known as macronutrients because the body needs them in large quantities. Vitamins and minerals are called micronutrients because they carry out specialized functions and are needed in smaller amounts. Your body also needs plenty of water.

Protein is the major component of muscles, organs, bones, skin, antibodies, some hormones, and most enzymes. Protein makes up nearly 25 percent of the typical American diet, more than twice the recommended 12 percent to 15 percent.

Carbohydrates are the body's main source of energy. Both simple (sugar) and complex (starch) carbohydrates are easily digested and converted into glucose, the main fuel for the body. However, complex carbohydrates are absorbed more slowly, while simple carbohydrates are quickly and easily absorbed. Any glucose not burned for immediate energy will be stored as fat. Foods rich in complex carbohydrates generally contain more vitamins, minerals, and fiber.

Dietary fiber may help lower your blood pressure, possibly by decreasing the amount of insulin circulating in the blood. It may also help the body get rid of more sodium. Insoluble fiber (fiber that is not broken down in the digestive tract) acts like a broom, pushing wastes through the digestive tract. Soluble fiber (fiber that is partially broken down in the digestive tract) seems to trap cholesterol (in bile, a substance produced by the liver and released in the small intestine during digestion) like a sponge.

There are three types of dietary fat: saturated, polyunsaturated, and monounsaturated. Most fatty foods contain a mixture of saturated and unsaturated fat. Eating too much of any type of fat will lead to weight gain, since all types of fat have the same amount of calories. Eating excessive amounts of saturated fat in particular will increase your chances of developing cancer, heart disease, diabetes, and other health problems. Eating too much saturated fat will also raise the level of cholesterol in your blood. Saturated fat should account for less than 10 percent of all calories consumed, and total fat in the diet should make up less than 30 percent of calories eaten per day.

Polyunsaturated fat, such as that found in vegetable oils and some fish, is less likely to raise cholesterol levels but can still contribute to weight gain. However, some polyunsaturated fats have an unusual chemical structure caused by food processing, such as when vegetable shortening or margarine are manufactured. These are called trans-fatty acids, and some research suggests that these altered vegetable fats are as bad for you as saturated fats. Monounsaturated fat, such as that found in olive oil, does not appear to cause any health problems when used in moderation. Though the evidence is still unclear, monounsaturated fat may even improve your heart's health.

Cholesterol is a lipid (a fatlike substance) found only in animal products. Although cholesterol is essential for many body processes, such as nerve function and cell reproduction, the body can manufacture all the cholesterol it needs. Most Americans eat considerably more than the recommended limit of 300 milligrams per day. All cholesterol that you eat is turned into some form of "bad" cholesterol, such as low density lipoprotein (LDL) cholesterol. LDL and other unhealthy types of cholesterol collect on the inside lining of your blood vessels. The "good" cholesterol, high density lipoprotein (HDL) cholesterol, is formed only in your body. You do not eat any HDL cholesterol in your diet. The HDL cholesterol is a larger particle and helps to remove fat from the blood and from the walls of your arteries.

Among the dozens of nutrients needed by the body for good health, some may be more important in blood pressure control than others, scientists have noticed. Sodium, of course, is the most widely publicized nutrient involved in high blood pressure. Sodium, with potassium, regulates the amount of water in the cells of the body. Sodium is also essential for the transmission of nerve impulses and the contraction of muscles. Potassium is essential for muscle contraction and other body functions. Potassium also plays a role in helping the kidneys eliminate sodium from the body. Some secondary causes of hypertension also cause hypokalemia, low blood levels of potassium.

Calcium is best known for providing the hard structure of bones and teeth. Calcium also plays an important role in the cardiovascular system. It is needed for proper blood clotting, and it helps maintain blood pressure by controlling contraction of the muscles in the heart and blood vessels. Magnesium is used by enzymes in the body responsible for storing and releasing energy from foods. Magnesium is needed for muscle contraction and for maintaining the proper level of calcium in the blood.

Because all these nutrients contribute in some way to the control of blood pressure, researchers have studied whether eating more or less of them helps people with hypertension.

THE FOOD GUIDE PYRAMID
To help you follow a healthy diet, the USDA developed the Food Guide Pyramid. The USDA recommends that about 60 percent of your calories come from carbohydrates, 30 percent from fat, and 10 percent from protein. The Food Guide Pyramid translates these percentages into servings of specific types of food.

The Food Guide Pyramid is designed to help you better understand which foods you need, from which groups, and in what amounts. What counts as one serving? **Milk, Yogurt, and Cheese Group:** 1 cup of milk or yogurt; 1½ to 2 ounces of cheese. **Meat,**

DIETARY GUIDELINES FOR AMERICANS

The Dietary Guidelines for Americans were developed through the joint efforts of the US Department of Agriculture (USDA) and the US Department of Health and Human Services (USDHHS). By following these helpful suggestions, you can improve your overall health and lower your risk of developing hypertension, heart disease, stroke, diabetes, and certain forms of cancer. These guidelines are geared toward healthy people aged 2 years and older:

- Eat a variety of foods.
- Maintain a healthy weight.
- Choose a diet low in total fat, saturated fat, and cholesterol.
- Choose a diet with plenty of vegetables, fruits, and whole-grain foods.
- Use sugar only in moderation.
- Use salt (sodium) only in moderation.
- If you drink alcohol, drink in moderation.

Poultry, Fish, Dry Beans, Eggs, and Nuts Group: 2 to 3 ounces of meat, fish, or poultry; ½ cup of cooked dry beans; 1 egg; 2 tablespoons of peanut butter. **Vegetable Group:** 1 cup of raw leafy vegetables; ½ cup of chopped raw or cooked vegetables; ¾ cup of vegetable juice. **Fruit Group:** 1 piece of fresh fruit or melon wedge; ½ cup of canned fruit; ½ cup of dried fruit; ¾ cup of fruit juice. **Bread, Cereal, Rice, and Pasta Group:** 1 slice of bread; 1 ounce of ready-to-eat cereal; ½ cup of cooked cereal, rice, or pasta.

The pyramid is based on an average 2,000-calorie-per-day diet. Depending on your activity level, you may need to take in more or less calories per day to maintain a healthy weight. In general, inactive women and older people need about 1,600 calories per day; children, teenage girls, active women, and inactive men should take in about 2,200 calories per day; and teenage boys, active men, and very active women need about 2,800 calories per day. If you are not sure how many calories you need, talk to your doctor.

Is Salt Important?

In some people, salt intake is linked directly to hypertension, stroke, and kidney function. A study of 10,000 men and women in 32 countries found that people who eat more salt are more likely to have high blood pressure. The amount of calcium lost through the urine is also higher in people who consume large

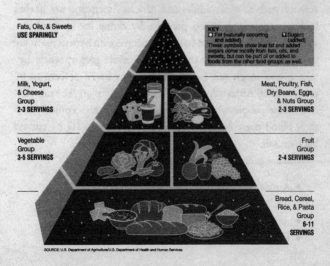

SOURCE: U.S. Department of Agriculture/U.S. Department of Health and Human Services

amounts of salt. Salt intake, no matter what the blood pressure, is an important independent predictor of left ventricular hypertrophy (see Chapter 3); even a moderate reduction in salt intake will reduce the size of the left ventricle. People with normal blood pressure are also likely to lower their systolic blood pressure and possibly, though to a lesser degree, diastolic blood pressure if they cut back on salt. The National Heart, Lung, and Blood Institute (NHLBI) has predicted that if everyone in the US ate 1 less teaspoon of salt each day, the rate of stroke would drop by 11 percent, heart attacks by 7 percent, and premature death due to disease by 5 percent.

Although it seems that everyone would be healthier if they took in less sodium, not everyone who has hypertension would experience a significant decrease in blood pressure on a low-sodium diet. As explained in Chapter 4, people with low renin activity, such as older adults and African Americans, are likelier to lower their high blood pressure by eating less sodium. Researchers think that about half of all people with hypertension are salt sensitive. This means their blood pressure goes up when they take in too much salt (sodium). As many as 70 percent to 80 percent of all African Americans with hypertension are salt sensitive. Some people who are especially salt sensitive could reduce their blood pressure by as much as 5 to 10 mm Hg by cutting back on salt.

You are more likely to be salt sensitive if you:

- Are an older person
- Are African American
- Are overweight
- Have diabetes

The only way to know for sure whether you are salt sensitive is to lower your sodium intake and monitor the effect on your blood pressure. (You may want to talk with your doctor about trying a simple salt step test.) Of course, for all the reasons mentioned above, your overall health will benefit from a lower sodium intake even if you do not notice a drop in blood pressure. In addition, eating less salt may help your blood pressure drugs work better, so that you need less medication.

What is a healthy goal for limiting salt intake? Your body needs only about 200 milligrams of sodium per day. Doctors recommend limiting salt intake to less than 2,400 milligrams (about 1 teaspoonful) per day.

Salt substitutes in which the sodium is replaced by potassium may be a good choice if you do not have kidney problems. However, be sure to ask your doctor before switching to these substitutes. If you are taking diuretics, the combination of a diet low in sodium and high in potassium could cause some problems. Talk to your doctor before making any changes in your diet. You should not worry about limiting your salt intake if recently you have had the flu or another illness that has caused vomiting and diarrhea. When you have recovered from your illness, you can gradually reduce your salt intake again.

Although you might think that shaking less salt onto your food will be a big help, 75 percent to 80 percent of the sodium in your diet comes from prepared foods; only 10 percent of the salt you eat is added at the table or during cooking. You will cut back on sodium more significantly if you avoid eating too many processed foods, such as canned soups and vegetables, frozen dinners, and sauce and gravy mixes. Check the nutrition information label on food packages for sodium content or read the list of

FOODS HIGH IN SALT (SODIUM)

Avoid or cut down on these and other high-sodium foods and ingredients to reduce your overall intake of sodium. Be sure to check nutrition information labels, lists of ingredients, and recipes for hidden sodium.

- Biscuits
- Bouillon
- Canned soups and pasta dishes
- Canned tomato or vegetable juices
- Canned vegetables
- Cheese
- Corn chips
- Crackers (salted)
- Deli meats
- Fast foods
- Frozen dinners
- Ham
- Hot dogs
- Ketchup
- Mustard
- Pancakes
- Pastries
- Pickles
- Potato chips
- Pretzels (salted)
- Processed and prepared foods (sauces, soups, rice or pasta dishes, baking and dessert mixes)
- Sardines
- Sauerkraut
- Sausages
- Self-rising flour
- Smoked meat or fish
- Soy sauce

SALTY INGREDIENTS TO WATCH OUT FOR

- Baking powder
- Baking soda
- Disodium phosphate
- Monosodium glutamate (MSG)
- Salt
- Sodium alginate
- Sodium benzoate
- Sodium hydroxide
- Sodium nitrite
- Sodium propionate
- Sodium sulfite

ingredients for the following red flags: sodium, salt, soda, or Na (the chemical abbreviation for sodium). Avoiding fast foods and snack products as much as possible will reduce the amount of sodium, fat, and cholesterol in your diet. You will also find that many herbs and spices enhance the flavor of foods better than salt does. As with other lifestyle changes, gradual is best here. Gradually reduce the amount of salt you add to foods and recipes and experiment with alternative flavorings.

Cutting Back on Fat and Cholesterol

As you hear so often, it is vital to eat less fat and cholesterol. Fat is a necessary source of energy and various chemical compounds, and fat helps the body absorb and use fat-soluble nutrients, such as beta carotene and vitamins A, D, E, and K. When you eat too much of some nutrients, the body simply eliminates them in the urine. When you eat too much fat, though, the body stores it.

The excess fat transported through your blood can cause other health problems, such as atherosclerosis (see Chapter 3). Fat does not dissolve in water (or in blood) and in fact separates from it, much like oil rises to the surface of water. The body usually bundles fat in the form of triglycerides. Triglycerides, like cholesterol, are transported in the body by molecules called lipoproteins. You already know that too much of some lipoproteins, the LDLs, is bad for your health, while high levels of other lipoproteins, the HDLs, are good for your health. LDL carries about 60 percent to 70 percent of the total amount of cholesterol in your blood, while HDL carries only 20 percent to 30 percent. The rest is carried by even smaller molecules, called very low density lipoproteins (VLDLs). VLDL only carries about 10 percent to 15 percent of the total cholesterol in the blood, mainly cholesterol made in the liver rather than from food being digested.

In the recent past, doctors emphasized your total cholesterol level. They now prefer to compare the amount of HDL ("good") cholesterol to LDL ("bad") cholesterol when assessing heart health. By monitoring the proportion of these molecules in your blood, your doctor can estimate your risk for heart disease. Many large medical studies have shown that having too little HDL and too much LDL indicates a high risk for heart disease, heart attack, and other health problems. Eating less cholesterol and less saturated fat is important for improving your cholesterol levels.

Eating less fat and cholesterol is more important for improving your overall cardiovascular health than for treating your hypertension. Researchers have not found a direct link between dietary fat and blood pressure. However, results of some studies have shown that eating less saturated fat and more fiber lowers blood pressure levels. In one study, men and women changed the amount and type of fat in their usual diet. They kept their body weight and sodium consumption constant while eating less fat (25 percent of total calories versus the 36 percent consumed by most Americans). They also ate more polyunsaturated fats and less saturated fats. As a result, they were able to lower their systolic and diastolic blood pressure levels an average of 9 percent. Not surprisingly, a diet low in sodium and low in fat was associated with greater reductions in blood pressure than either a low-sodium or low-fat diet alone. When changing the fat content of your diet, remember that saturated fat is found mainly in animal products, such as butter, whole milk, red meat, and lard, and in many baked goods.

Other Healthful Changes to Your Diet

Eating a well-balanced diet can help maintain good health and reduce your risk of most chronic diseases, such as heart disease, cancer, osteoporosis, and diabetes. Researchers have identified specific nutrients as important to specific aspects of health. As noted earlier in the chapter, calcium, potassium, magnesium, and fish oil have all been examined for their role in blood pressure control.

Medical studies that follow large groups of people over time, matching what they eat with specific health measures, have noted that people who consume a lot of calcium usually have normal blood pressure. Levels of calcium in the blood are lower among people with hypertension who also have low renin activity (see Chapter 4). Calcium levels are higher among those people with high renin activity than in people with normal blood pressure or other people with hypertension. If you have low renin activity or know that you are salt sensitive, you may benefit from eating more calcium. If this is difficult because of lactose intolerance, you can take calcium supplements or drink orange juice fortified with calcium. Since most Americans do not get enough calcium in their diets, eating more low-fat dairy products, green leafy vegetables, and other foods rich in calcium is a good idea for most people. However, eating a high-calcium diet does not affect your need to take blood pressure medication.

Studies of large groups have found that people who take in a lot of potassium tend to have low blood pressure, as do those who have a high calcium intake. Clinical studies testing specific treatments of hypertension suggest that potassium supplements can reduce blood pressure, particularly in people who have a diet high in sodium. Studies in animals also suggest that this extra potassium may protect against strokes. The amount of potassium in the diet may be particularly important for people taking certain diuretic drugs (see Chapter 8) that can cause the kidneys to eliminate too much potassium.

However, you should be careful about using potassium supplements if you have diabetes or kidney disease or are taking potassium-sparing diuretics, angiotensin converting enzyme (ACE) inhibitors (see Chapter 9), or nonsteroidal anti-inflammatory drugs (NSAIDs, such as aspirin, ibuprofen, and most other nonprescription pain relievers). Excessive amounts of potassium can be dangerous in older adults, too, because older people cannot eliminate the additional potassium as quickly as younger people can. The extra potassium can interfere with a normal heartbeat, causing arrhythmia. In any case, you will enjoy other health benefits by eating a variety of foods rich in potassium (see page 99) instead of taking potassium supplements.

FOODS RICH IN POTASSIUM

Add these potassium-rich foods to your diet to make sure you get enough potassium every day:

- Apples
- Apricots
- Asparagus
- Bananas
- Broccoli
- Cabbage
- Cantaloupe
- Cauliflower
- Chicken
- Dried figs
- Dried peas and beans
- Eggplant
- Lean red meat
- Molasses
- Nectarines
- Nonfat and low-fat dairy products
- Orange juice
- Oranges
- Potatoes
- Prunes
- Raisins
- Reduced-fat peanut butter
- Squash
- Sweet potatoes
- Tomatoes
- Watermelon

Magnesium is another nutrient that may be linked to blood pressure. Researchers have noted that people who take in more magnesium tend to have lower blood pressure. However, clinical trials testing magnesium as a possible treatment for hypertension have not yet reported any improvement in people taking magnesium supplements.

You have probably heard that eating fish twice a week is good for your heart, and indeed it is. In some studies, eating fish or taking fish-oil capsules appeared to be associated with a reduction in blood pressure—a reduction of from 3 to 6 mm Hg in systolic pressure and of from 2 to 4 mm Hg in diastolic pressure. In other studies, however, researchers were disappointed by the apparent lack of effect fish consumption had on blood pressure. In any case, bake or steam your fish; frying eliminates these potential health benefits.

Other dietary changes also have been shown to lower blood pressure, though these have not been thoroughly studied. Eating a vegetarian diet, eating more fiber (especially soluble fiber), and eating less protein (especially if the kidneys have been damaged by high blood pressure) may help with your blood pressure management. Vegetarians tend to have lower blood pressure levels and a lower risk of developing hypertension than do nonvegetarians. Compared with the nonvegetarian diet, the vegetarian diet contains more polyunsaturated fat, fiber, vegetable protein, potassium, and magnesium and less total fat, saturated fat, cholesterol, and vitamin B_{12}. Eating at least five servings of vegetables and fruits per day will also supply plenty of antioxidants (such as vitamins A, C, and E), substances that reduce the amount of damage to the inner lining of the arteries and slow the progress of atherosclerosis (see Chapter 3).

Finally, drinking caffeinated beverages will raise your blood pressure in the short run but probably will not contribute to your hypertension. However, be sure to avoid consuming anything that contains caffeine before having your blood pressure checked.

LIMIT ALCOHOL USE

Alcohol consumption raises blood pressure both in the short term and in the long term. In fact, alcohol is known to have a greater effect on blood pressure than salt. In the Framingham Heart Study, evidence showed that increases in blood pressure are directly related to the amount of alcohol consumed. In other words, drinking more alcohol leads to higher blood pressure.

Alcohol can affect blood pressure in anyone who drinks regularly, but its effects are particularly noticeable in overweight people and older adults. People who are stressed may also be prone to the blood pressure–raising effects of alcohol. Risk of alcohol-induced hypertension is higher among people who take in a lot of sodium or who are not physically active. Higher rates of hemorrhagic stroke (when a blood vessel bursts and leaks blood into the brain) have been found in heavy drinkers.

It is a good idea to limit yourself to two drinks per day: two 12-ounce beers, two 4-ounce glasses of wine, or two mixed drinks. After you reach your limit, drink soft drinks, juice, or water.

The bottom line: if you drink alcohol, do so in moderation. If you are taking any medication, be sure to ask your doctor or pharmacist about possible interactions between alcohol and the drugs you take.

STOP SMOKING

Chemicals in tobacco smoke damage the lining of your arteries and make them more susceptible to the buildup of plaque. This, combined with the force of high blood pressure, is likely to cause serious damage to your blood vessels. The nicotine in tobacco is a powerful stimulant that also affects your heart and blood vessels. When you smoke or chew tobacco, your heart beats faster, your arteries constrict, and your blood pressure shoots up. Smoking is also associated with an increase in total and LDL ("bad") cholesterol and a decrease in HDL ("good") cholesterol. Smokeless tobacco contains nicotine, sodium, and natural licorice, all of which contribute to high blood pressure. (See box, How to Quit Smoking, on page 103).

REDUCE STRESS IN YOUR LIFE

There is no conclusive scientific evidence that stress causes hypertension. However, it has been shown that stress can make hypertension more difficult to manage. When faced with stress, your heart rate increases and your blood vessels constrict, raising your blood pressure. You may be able to lower your blood pressure by reducing stress in your life.

Before you can take steps to reduce stress, you need to determine the cause. Stress is caused by both negative and positive situations. What is stressful for one person may not be stressful for another. And keep in mind that you may not always be able to avoid or eliminate every possible source of stress in your life.

HOW TO QUIT SMOKING

- Choose a day to quit, and quit on that day.
- Share the news with your friends and family; they will be a good source of support in the weeks ahead.
- Dispose of all smoking materials (including cigarettes, matches, lighters, and ashtrays) you have kept at home, at work, and in your car.
- Avoid situations that may encourage you to smoke (for example, do not sit in the smoking section of restaurants).
- If you crave a cigarette, use sugarless gum or hard candies as a smoking substitute.
- Drink at least eight glasses of water, 8 ounces each, every day.
- Snack on fresh fruit and raw vegetables.
- Ask your doctor for advice about using a nicotine patch or nicotine gum.
- Join a quit-smoking support group.

DEEP BREATHING EXERCISES

Deep breathing is one of the easiest ways to relax and reduce stress. You can do it just about anywhere, anytime. Try this whenever you feel tense. Stop if you start to feel dizzy.

- Sit or lie in a comfortable position with your eyes closed.
- Relax all of your muscles and concentrate on your breathing.
- Breathe in and out through your nose.
- Breathe deeply, pulling air deep into your lungs.
- Exhale completely, breathing out as much air as possible before taking your next breath.
- Continue breathing deeply for 5 to 10 minutes.
- When finished, remain quiet with your eyes closed for a few more minutes, then open your eyes slowly.

Here are some common sources of stress:

- A new baby
- Moving to a new home
- Death of a friend or family member
- Marital problems
- Illness of a friend or family member
- Problems at work
- Job change or job loss
- Retirement (you or your spouse)
- Change in financial status (for better or worse)
- Sexual problems
- Personal illness or injury

Here are some useful tips for dealing with stress:

- Find time to relax; take time for yourself.
- Live in the present; you cannot change the past and you cannot control the future.
- Eat a well-balanced diet; include plenty of fruits and vegetables.
- Exercise regularly; aerobic exercise is best.
- Set priorities; complete tasks and solve problems one at a time.
- Stay active and focused; keep busy doing things you enjoy.
- Get plenty of rest; get a good night's sleep every night.
- Talk your problems over with someone you can trust.
- See your doctor if you feel overwhelmed and unable to cope; he or she will be able to recommend an appropriate support group or therapist.

HOW TO GET A GOOD NIGHT'S SLEEP

Getting plenty of sleep will help to lower your blood pressure. Here are some steps you can take if you are having problems getting to sleep at night:

- Exercise moderately during the day so that you will feel tired at bedtime (but avoid exercising right before bedtime).
- Go to bed and get up at about the same time every day (and avoid napping during the day).
- A warm bath and a warm glass of (low-fat) milk may help you to relax.
- If you read in bed, choose something light or soothing.
- Be sure your mattress and pillows are comfortable.
- For an ideal room temperature for sleeping, keep the thermostat set between 60 and 65 degrees Fahrenheit.
- If you are still awake, get up and do a couple of light chores or some light reading until you feel sleepy.

7

Medication for Hypertension

For some people, making lifestyle changes (see Chapter 6) will be enough to maintain a healthy blood pressure level. For others, drugs are needed to control the dangerous effects of hypertension. Whether drugs are necessary is often decided by your genes—a risk factor that you cannot control.

With other medical conditions, people who must use medication generally feel some relief or improvement after taking the drugs. For example, aspirin can relieve pain, and antibiotics, a bacterial infection. However, since you probably do not have any symptoms directly related to your high blood pressure, you will probably not feel different after taking medication. Blood pressure medications are prescribed to prevent future and possibly severe health problems, not to relieve symptoms. The benefits of blood pressure medications have been proved in many studies. In general, people with hypertension who use medication to control their blood pressure have a lower risk of heart attack and stroke.

Because of unpleasant drug side effects, it used to be said about hypertension that the treatment was worse than the disease. Today, this is no longer true. Medications designed to control blood pressure have come a long way. Drug companies have developed products that lower blood pressure while causing fewer unpleasant side effects. One very large study showed that people who took any of five different blood pressure–lowering medications felt better after they started drug treatment than they had before treatment. The researchers asked about energy level, mood, general health, satisfaction with health, and whether the drugs interfered with daily routine. People taking any of the active drugs reported fewer problems than those taking the placebo (an inactive pill given instead of a real drug to test the drug's effectiveness).

However, you may still experience some unpleasant effects related to your medication. If so, you should discuss these side effects with your physician. Never stop taking your medication unless told to do so by your doctor. Even if you do not have a problem with side effects, your doctor may want to monitor other health risk factors, such as your blood cholesterol level. Because so many drugs are available, your doctor can work with you to ensure that you get the best treatment with the fewest side effects and risks.

Because drug costs can account for 70 percent to 80 percent of the cost of treating hypertension, most doctors weigh the specific benefits of a particular medication against its cost before making a decision. If you are concerned about the cost of your medication, be sure to talk with your physician or pharmacist about possible less expensive alternatives. For some medications, you may be able to use a generic version or substitute an equivalent drug; for others, you may need to take exactly what your doctor has prescribed. Sometimes a change as simple as prescribing a higher-dose pill (which you can then break in half) can lower costs significantly.

STARTING YOUR MEDICATION

Unless your hypertension is especially severe or complicated by other health problems, you will probably start with just one anti-hypertensive medication. Most doctors start with diuretics, beta blockers, or calcium channel blockers (see Chapters 8 and 9). Some people, however, do better starting with an angiotensin converting enzyme (ACE) inhibitor (Chapter 9), especially if they have diabetes or high renin activity. Alpha blockers, angiotensin II blockers (see Chapter 9), and other supplemental drugs (see Chapter 10) may be used as a second medication to improve the effectiveness of the first medication selected or in special situations.

Most blood pressure medications are taken once a day. They typically start to work 1 to 2 hours after they are taken and have their greatest effect 4 to 6 hours after they are taken. Most people take their medication in the morning. Whenever you take your medication, be sure to make it part of your daily routine (such as when you eat breakfast) so that you will remember to take it.

When you first start drug therapy, your doctor will want to check your blood pressure and general health at regular intervals.

If you have mild hypertension with no complications, he or she may wait as long as 1 to 2 months. The results of the examinations, laboratory tests, and blood pressure monitoring will help your doctor decide how frequently to see you. If you experience any unpleasant side effects, you should always call your doctor right away. Once your blood pressure is stabilized, you will probably need to see your doctor every 3 to 6 months, depending on your general health and response to treatment.

CHANGES IN MEDICATION

Sometimes one medication does not control your blood pressure as well as your doctor thought it would. Because you will start with the lowest recommended dose for your drug, your doctor will wait several weeks to give your first medication time to take effect. He or she may then increase the dose to the next recommended level.

If 2 to 3 months have passed with no significant benefit, your doctor will decide whether to try a higher dose for your current medication, to prescribe an additional drug, or to switch you to a different single medication. Results from a large study conducted by the Veterans Affairs Cooperative Study Group on Antihypertensive Agents suggest that it is better to switch to a different single drug treatment than to add another drug to the regimen. In this study, of those whose first drug failed, 49 percent reached their blood pressure goal with the second single drug.

On the other hand, combining antihypertensive medications may allow you to take smaller doses of each drug, which should lessen your chances of experiencing unpleasant side effects.

WHEN DRUGS DO NOT WORK

You will work closely with your doctor to develop a medication treatment plan that works best for you. However, if the drugs are not helping, you may want to consider the following possible causes of ineffective drug treatment. If you think any of these factors could be interfering with your drug therapy, be sure to tell your doctor.

- Medication causes unpleasant or embarrassing side effects
- Medication is too expensive (taking only part of a dose or skipping doses)
- Instructions for taking medication not clear
- Medication is inconvenient to take
- Forget to take medication
- Not happy with medication choice
- Weight gain
- Drinking alcohol
- Smoking cigarettes
- Chewing tobacco
- Taking other drugs that may interfere:
  - Nonsteroidal anti-inflammatory drugs (NSAIDs, such as aspirin or other pain-killers)
  - Oral contraceptives
  - Sympathomimetics (such as epinephrine, norepinephrine, appetite suppressants, asthma and allergy medications, cold remedies, and nasal decongestants)
  - Antidepressants
  - Cyclosporine
  - Erythropoietin
  - Cocaine

Sometimes you can eventually stop taking one of the medications. Taking just one medication is usually easier and less expensive, and your doctor will want to do everything he or she can to help you stick with your drug treatment plan.

Once you have a drug treatment plan that controls your blood pressure, there is usually no reason to change the plan later. Most medications work indefinitely. However, you may develop other health problems that may cause your doctor to consider changing your drug treatment plan.

If your blood pressure is especially high or if you have damage to certain organs caused by your high blood pressure, your doctor may not want to wait before changing your medication. In these situations, getting your blood pressure under control is the top priority. You may need to take two or even three drugs until your doctor is satisfied that you are no longer at risk for serious, perhaps life-threatening health problems. Once your blood pressure is under control, your doctor may work with you to reduce the number or dose of your medications.

Some drug combinations are better than others in certain circumstances. Taking a diuretic and a calcium channel blocker lowers blood pressure through two complementary methods: reducing blood volume and dilating (widening) blood vessels. A more potent combination for lowering blood pressure pairs a calcium channel blocker with an ACE inhibitor. For people who also have angina (chest pain), hypertension may respond to a calcium channel blocker with a beta blocker. Some medications are available that combine two types of drugs in one pill.

After your blood pressure has been stable for at least 1 year, your doctor may consider trying step-down therapy to reduce or eliminate your medications. Of course, to consider this option,

CATEGORIES OF ANTIHYPERTENSIVE DRUGS

TYPE OF DRUG	METHOD OF ACTION	USEFUL FOR . . .	NOT GOOD FOR . . .	SIDE EFFECTS
Diuretics	Reduce salt and water in the body	African Americans, older adults, people with heart failure or low renin activity	People with diabetes, gout, or high renin activity; women with preeclampsia	Low potassium levels, muscle cramps, fatigue, weakness, impotence
Beta blockers	Slow heart rate and block renin output by kidneys	People recovering from heart attack; people with high renin activity, high resting heart rate, enlarged heart, angina, coronary artery disease, or migraine headache; younger adults	People with asthma, heart failure, chronic obstructive pulmonary disease, peripheral vascular disease, insulin-dependent diabetes, or Raynaud's syndrome; athletic people; people with depression	Bronchospasm (like an asthma attack), fatigue, insomnia, impotence, reduced exercise tolerance
Angiotensin converting enzyme (ACE) inhibitors	Prevent arteries from constricting	People with diabetes, congestive heart failure, high renin activity, or certain kidney diseases	People with renal artery blockage, abnormal kidney function, or only one kidney; pregnant women	Cough, skin rash, elevated potassium levels

Calcium channel blockers	Relax arterial walls	African Americans; older adults; people with angina, arrhythmia, diabetes, Raynaud's syndrome, migraine, or pulmonary hypertension	People with left ventricular dysfunction, liver disease, or heart failure	Constipation, ankle swelling, headache, flushing, changes in the gums, rapid heartbeat
Alpha blockers	Prevent arteries from constricting	People with high cholesterol levels, diabetes, peripheral vascular disease, or chronic obstructive pulmonary disease	People with postural hypotension, depression, or enlarged heart	Dramatic initial drop in blood pressure (fainting), stuffy nose, skin rash, headache, dizziness, weakness, mild fluid retention
Angiotensin blockers	Prevent arteries from constricting, prevent kidneys from retaining salt and water	People who cannot tolerate ACE inhibitors	Pregnant women	Fatigue, stomach pain
Centrally acting drugs	Lower heart rate and peripheral resistance through actions on the brain and nerves		Older adults; people with liver disease or depression	Drowsiness, dry mouth, fatigue, postural hypotension, sexual dysfunction, severe withdrawal syndrome
Direct vasodilators	Relax arterial walls	Only used in people whose blood pressure cannot be controlled with other drugs and in emergencies		Rapid heart rate, palpitations, fluid retention, headache, stuffy nose, nausea, fatigue

you must be prepared to stick with the important lifestyle changes you have already made: weight control, exercise, healthy diet, alcohol only in moderation, and no smoking. If these healthful habits are not firmly in place, you probably will not be able to cut back on your medication.

Any reduction in your blood pressure medication must be done gradually, with your doctor's supervision. You will need to monitor your blood pressure at home, and you will need to schedule regular follow-up visits with your doctor. Even if you can maintain normal blood pressure without medication, you will still need to see your doctor as often as he or she recommends and monitor your blood pressure between visits.

OVERVIEW OF BLOOD PRESSURE MEDICATIONS

The next three chapters review currently available antihypertensive medications in detail. You may find it useful to learn a little about each of the major types of drugs. This will help you understand why your doctor chose the medication he or she did, and why the drug your friend is using might not work for you. The table on pages 112 through 113 summarizes the main types of antihypertensive drugs, their method of lowering blood pressure, the people they are most likely to help, the people who probably or definitely should not use them, and their major side effects. You can use the index of this book to locate names of medications you are taking for hypertension and then refer back to this table. The table may be especially useful if you have questions about a drug you heard or read about. For example, you may want to know why you cannot take a particular medication.

8

Choices for Initial
Drug Therapy

As discussed in Chapter 7, several factors govern which drugs
might be appropriate for your treatment. Usually, in cases of mild
hypertension with no other risks, your doctor will prescribe a
diuretic, a beta blocker, or a calcium channel blocker. In some
cases, the doctor may prescribe a combination drug (see
page 129).

DIURETICS

No simpler, more cost-effective antihypertensive drug exists than
a diuretic, often called a "water pill." Thiazide diuretics effectively
lower blood pressure in all groups, especially African Americans
and older adults. They are inexpensive and generally well toler-

ated. Diuretics are a logical second drug when combination therapy is needed. They are usually effective within 3 to 4 days.

Diuretics work by preventing the reabsorption of salt and water from urine by the kidneys. The amount of urine increases, and the amount of salt and water in the body decreases. The result is similar to being on a low-sodium diet. Cardiac output (the amount of blood your heart pumps) goes down initially, followed by a reduction in total peripheral resistance (the degree to which blood vessels resist blood flow). Both changes contribute to the drop in blood pressure. This action by diuretics can make them useful in treating hypertension in people who also have heart or kidney failure.

Three types of diuretics are available. Thiazide diuretics are the most common type and are usually what doctors mean when they refer to diuretics. Loop diuretics have the same general effect as thiazide diuretics but have a slightly different method for increasing urine output. Potassium-sparing diuretics are newer and were developed to prevent excess loss of potassium in the urine.

For a long time, diuretics were the only medication available for treating hypertension. Doctors now know that certain people will do better using diuretics than other drugs, such as people with low renin activity. Conversely, people with an active renin system will not benefit as much from diuretics because their kidneys will produce additional renin. This extra renin in turn will cause the kidneys to retain sodium in exchange for potassium, canceling out the effect of the diuretic. Thiazide diuretics should be used cautiously by people with diabetes, with a history of gout, or with hypercalcemia (too much calcium in the blood). Cholesterol levels may rise initially in people taking a diuretic, but research has shown that these elevations disappear within a year.

Anyone with an enlarged heart and any pregnant woman diagnosed with preeclampsia (see Chapter 12) should not take diuretics.

Diuretics may not work as well when other medications are also taken. Cholestyramine and colestipol (both used to lower blood cholesterol levels) can cause diuretics to be less effective. So can nonsteroidal anti-inflammatory drugs (NSAIDs), such as aspirin, ibuprofen, and other commonly used painkillers. Finally, diuretics can raise the level of lithium in patients using this medication.

All diuretics cause some increase in urination. Thiazide and loop diuretics, particularly when taken in high doses, lower the level of potassium in the body and produce significant hypokalemia (abnormally low levels of potassium in the blood) in some people. This can lead to arrhythmias and palpitations (an abnormally strong, rapid heartbeat). The most common side effects of diuretics are impotence, reduced libido, muscle cramps, and fatigue. Because diuretics interfere with the body's ability to remove uric acid, a waste product in the blood, some people who take these drugs develop gout, a condition in which uric acid accumulates in and inflames various joints. Use of diuretics can also lower the amount of magnesium in the body, which can contribute to an irregular heartbeat (as can low potassium). When blood levels of potassium are low, diuretics can raise blood sugar, possibly increasing the risk of diabetes.

The table on page 118 lists the class, brand, and chemical (or generic) names of some commonly used diuretics. The dose range shown is recommended by the Joint National Committee on Detection, Evaluation, and Treatment of High Blood Pressure; do not adjust the dose you are taking without talking to your doctor.

DIURETICS

CLASS	GENERIC NAME	BRAND NAME	ADULT DOSAGE (MILLIGRAMS/DAY)
Thiazides and related agents	Bendroflumethiazide	Naturetin	2.5 to 5.0
	Chlorothiazide	Diuril	125 to 500
	Chlorthalidone	Hygroton, Thalitone	12.5 to 50.0
	Hydrochlorothiazide	Esidrix, HydroDIURIL, Oretic	12.5 to 50.0
	Indapamide	Lozol	2.5 to 5.0
	Methylclothiazide	Enduron	2.5 to 5.0
	Metolazone	Zaroxolyn	0.5 to 5.0
Loop diuretics	Bumetanide	Bumex	0.5 to 5.0
	Ethacrynic acid	Edecrin	25 to 100
	Furosemide	Lasix	20 to 320
Potassium-sparing	Amiloride	Midamor	5 to 10
	Spironolactone	Aldactone	25 to 100
	Triamterene	Dyrenium	50 to 150

Recently, a new 12.5-milligram formulation of hydrochlorothiazide came on the market (brand name, Microzide). This convenient pill eliminates the need to break 25-milligram pills in half. Most of the thiazide diuretics are taken only once a day, but the loop diuretics and sometimes the potassium-sparing diuretics are taken twice a day.

BETA BLOCKERS

Like diuretics, beta blockers have been used for many years and have undergone extensive testing in clinical trials. Beta blockers were originally developed for treating heart disease, and their effect on blood pressure was noticed later. Beta blockers have been used effectively and safely in combination with all other types of antihypertensive drugs, though caution may be needed when combining them with a calcium channel blocker (see Chapter 9).

Beta blockers are a type of adrenergic inhibitor. That is, they interfere with uptake of norepinephrine (a hormone that constricts blood vessels and increases heart rate, thereby increasing blood pressure) from nerve cells. As the name implies, beta blockers block beta receptors on the surface of the heart, kidneys, blood vessels, and other tissues. These receptors normally receive chemical messages from norepinephrine and respond in ways that raise blood pressure (see Chapter 1). When beta blockers sit on the receptors on the heart, they slow heart rate and lower cardiac output. When they block receptors on the kidneys, they prevent renin production. Both actions help prevent increased blood pressure.

This type of activity can cause problems for people with asthma or other chronic obstructive pulmonary disease (COPD), since the response to beta blockers in the lungs is a slight constriction of airways. People with peripheral vascular disease may notice a worsening of constriction (and therefore pain) in the arteries of their legs. Athletic individuals will notice fatigue resulting from lower cardiac output and should consider taking a different type of drug. Beta blockers should be used with caution in people with type I (insulin-dependent) diabetes because they can mask the symptoms of and delay recovery from hypoglycemia (low blood sugar). Beta blockers also decrease high density lipoprotein (HDL, or "good") cholesterol and increase triglyceride levels.

People with high renin activity benefit more from beta blockers because of their effect on the release of renin by the kidneys. Beta blockers seem to be more effective at lowering blood pres-

119

sure in younger people than in older adults and in whites than in blacks. Because beta blockers are effective in treating angina, they are the drug of choice in people with known coronary artery disease. People who are recovering from a heart attack will also benefit from treatment with beta blockers. Not surprisingly, they are also the best drug for people with a rapid resting heart rate. People who have migraine headaches may also want to consider taking beta blockers because they prevent excessive dilation (widening) of arteries in the brain and its accompanying pain.

The most common adverse effects of beta blockers include a slow heartbeat, congestive heart failure in susceptible people, fatigue, and impotence. Switching to a different beta blocker may alleviate these symptoms.

Talk to your doctor or pharmacist about when to take your medication. Most of these drugs are taken once a day, but some are taken twice a day. Medications that combine a beta blocker with an alpha blocker are described in Chapter 9. Four of the beta blockers listed in the table on page 121 have what is known as intrinsic sympathomimetic activity. These drugs—acebutolol, carteolol, penbutolol, and pindolol—do not affect blood cholesterol levels and are less likely to slow the heart rate as much as the other beta blockers.

In the table on page 121, the dosage ranges recommended by the Joint National Committee on Detection, Evaluation, and Treatment of High Blood Pressure are provided along with the brand and chemical names of some commonly prescribed beta blockers. Do not change the dosage you are taking without talking to your doctor. In 1995, the US Food and Drug Administration (USFDA) approved a beta blocker with vasodilating effects (widens the blood vessels; see Chapter 10) called carvedilol

BETA BLOCKERS

GENERIC NAME	BRAND NAME	ADULT DOSAGE (MILLIGRAMS/DAY)
Acebutolol	Sectral	200 to 1,200
Atenolol	Tenormin	25 to 100
Betaxolol	Kerlone	5 to 40
Carteolol	Cartrol	2.5 to 10.0
Metoprolol	Lopressor	50 to 200
Metoprolol (extended release)	Toprol-XL	50 to 200
Nadolol	Corgard	20 to 240
Penbutolol	Levatol	20 to 80
Pindolol	Visken	10 to 60
Propranolol	Inderal	40 to 240
Propranolol (long acting)	Inderal LA	60 to 240
Timolol	Blocadren	20 to 40

(brand name, Coreg). Carvedilol can cause postural hypotension (abnormally low blood pressure that occurs when a person sits up or stands suddenly) and may interact with other drugs taken for heart conditions and with insulin. The starting dose is 12.5 milligrams per day (taken in two 6.25-milligram doses), though usually no more than 50 milligrams per day (two 25-milligram doses) are prescribed. Nebivolol and celiprolol are newer drugs that also offer both selective beta blocker activity and vasodilating effects.

CALCIUM CHANNEL BLOCKERS

Calcium channel blockers have been available in the US since the late 1970s. They are effective in reducing blood pressure in most people with hypertension and are prescribed as frequently as diuretics and angiotensin converting enzyme (ACE) inhibitors (see Chapter 9)—and more frequently than beta blockers. Like diuretics, they are particularly effective in African Americans and older adults. They have been used successfully in combination with all other types of antihypertensive drugs. The availability of sustained-release formulations (that is, pills that release the medication gradually over many hours) makes these drugs well tolerated and convenient for general use.

As explained in Chapter 1, contraction of the smooth muscles in arteries is triggered by calcium's entering the cells, which it does through special channels in cell membranes. Calcium channel blockers obstruct the entrance to these channels and thus weaken the contraction of the muscle cells, opening the arteries and lowering blood pressure. Calcium is not involved in the contraction of skeletal muscles, so no weakness occurs in these muscles. In animal studies, calcium channel blockers have also been noted to prevent the development of plaques (see Chapter 3). In humans, some evidence suggests that certain drugs (nifedipine and nicardipine) may slow or block the development of plaques in the coronary arteries. Some calcium channel blockers (verapamil and diltiazem) slow the heart rate and the conduction of electrical signals through heart tissues, making them useful for people with arrhythmias.

On the other hand, verapamil should not be used by people who have left ventricular dysfunction (often characterized by a low level of blood pumped out of the heart to the body). It should also be used cautiously by people who have arrhythmias. Calcium channel blockers are removed from the blood by the liver, so they should be used carefully in people with liver disease.

People with angina (chest pain) will gain extra benefit from calcium channel blockers, since their coronary arteries will be dilated, reducing the amount and frequency of pain. People with diabetes may also do well with calcium channel blockers, since these drugs do not worsen glucose intolerance or cholesterol levels and may slow the rate of decline in kidney function. People who need to take NSAIDs regularly may do better with calcium channel blockers than other types of antihypertensive medication because the two drugs do not interfere with each other.

Calcium channel blockers have gained tremendous popularity because they have very few side effects. In fact, in studies that compared several types of antihypertensive drugs, they were the best tolerated. However, calcium channel blockers can cause constipation because the intestines have the same type of smooth muscle (requiring calcium to contract) as the arteries. Other possible side effects include swelling of the ankles, headache, flushing, dizziness, and changes in the gums.

The results of one study suggested that people who take the calcium channel blockers nisoldipine, felodipine, nifedipine, verapamil, or diltiazem should avoid grapefruit and grapefruit juice. Because grapefruit contains a substance that blocks the specific enzyme responsible for breaking down these calcium channel blockers, it may cause the drug to accumulate in the blood. When blood levels of the drug get too high, such side effects as palpitations, headache, ankle swelling, and angina can occur. Some calcium channel blockers, especially those in extended-release forms, should not be taken with a high-fat meal, since this combination may speed delivery of the drug to the body.

Verapamil and some other calcium channel blockers can

increase blood levels of certain drugs: digoxin, carbamazepine, prazosin, quinidine, theophylline, and cyclosporine. The effectiveness of verapamil can be affected by certain medications as well. Be sure to ask your doctor or pharmacist about drug interactions if you are taking a calcium channel blocker with any other medication.

Some calcium channel blockers are available in fast, short-acting versions used in emergency situations (see Chapter 11). These short-acting calcium channel blockers can cause unpleasant and possibly dangerous side effects—including heart attack and angina—and should not be used in the long-term management of hypertension. Doctors instead prescribe the extended-release versions of these drugs, which allow the medication to be released slowly and over a long period of time. None of the serious side effects associated with the short-acting versions have been seen in the extended-release pills.

Calcium channel blockers can be used in combination with beta blockers, ACE inhibitors, and diuretics. People whose condition has responded poorly to a single drug even at the highest dose may benefit from the addition of a calcium channel blocker to their treatment.

The table on page 125 lists the dosage range recommended by the Joint National Committee on Detection, Evaluation, and Treatment of High Blood Pressure for some commonly prescribed calcium channel blockers. Do not change the dosage you are taking without talking to your doctor. A newer calcium channel blocker, Tiazac, has been approved as a sustained-release (and less expensive) version of diltiazem (also available as Cardizem and Dilacor). Tiazac contains a high concentration of diltiazem beads that are released at a smooth and steady rate. This ensures

CALCIUM CHANNEL BLOCKERS

GENERIC NAME	BRAND NAME	ADULT DOSAGE (MILLIGRAMS/DAY)
Amlodipine	Norvasc	2.5 to 10.0
Diltiazem	Cardizem	90 to 360
Diltiazem (sustained release)	Cardizem SR	120 to 360
Diltiazem (extended release)	Dilacor XR	180 to 360
Felodipine (sustained release)	Plendil Extended Release	5 to 10
Isradipine	DynaCirc	2.5 to 10.0
Nicardipine (sustained release)	Cardene SR	60 to 120
Nifedipine	Adalat, Procardia	30 to 120
Nifedipine (sustained release)	Adalat CC, Procardia XL	30 to 90
Verapamil	Calan, Isoptin	80 to 360
Verapamil (long acting)	Calan SR, Isoptin SR, Verelan	120 to 360

that blood pressure remains level over the entire 24-hour period. Another newer calcium channel blocker, Sular (nisoldipine), is chemically similar to several other available drugs in this group (such as nifedipine). It is less expensive and provides smooth, continuous control of blood pressure.

Other extended-release versions of calcium channel blockers are now available. Covera-HS is a once-daily, controlled-release formulation of verapamil. The delivery system has two stages. First, it provides a 4- to 5-hour drug release so that, when taken at bedtime, peak levels of medication coincide with waking and the first hours of activity. Second, the extended release of the drug in the digestive tract provides 24-hour control of blood pressure and angina.

Finally, new calcium channel blockers may be on the market soon. Lacidipine (the generic name) has proved to be an effective and well-tolerated drug in almost 19,000 people with hypertension who have participated in early drug trials. In Europe, manidipine has also proved to be safe and effective.

9

Other Drug Options

Researchers have been working to identify ways to lower blood pressure without interfering with other body functions. Because so many organ systems are involved in controlling blood pressure, this has proved difficult. All of the drugs reviewed in this chapter lower blood pressure effectively. Some offer special benefits to certain people, and most have fewer side effects. However, these drugs come at quite a price: they are much more expensive than either diuretics or generic beta blockers. Since patients with hypertension must often be treated for their entire lifetime, cost is an important concern. In addition, because these drugs are newer, the effects of their use over 10, 20, 30, or more years remain unknown. Researchers are especially interested to learn whether they reduce the risk of heart attack and stroke.

ANGIOTENSIN CONVERTING ENZYME INHIBITORS

Angiotensin converting enzyme (ACE) inhibitors lower blood pressure in all types of people with hypertension, including older adults. African Americans are generally less sensitive to the antihypertensive effects of ACE inhibitors than are whites, but increasing the dose or adding a diuretic eliminates this difference.

As explained in Chapter 1, ACE is an enzyme that triggers the conversion of an inactive substance, angiotensin I, into a powerful substance that constricts arteries, angiotensin II. ACE inhibitors inactivate this enzyme and thus reduce the amount of angiotensin II in the blood. With less angiotensin II acting on the arteries, they can expand, thereby lowering blood pressure.

ACE inhibitors are the drugs of choice in hypertensive people who have congestive heart failure and are also useful for people with diabetes who also have kidney problems. ACE inhibitors work best in people who have high renin activity. They also can be used in treating renovascular hypertension (see Chapter 2). However, in people with only one kidney, with blockage of both renal arteries, or with a transplanted kidney affected by renal artery blockage, ACE inhibition may contribute to kidney failure. In addition, pregnant women and women who are trying to become pregnant should avoid ACE inhibitors.

ACE inhibitors are generally free from many of the side effects, such as fatigue and impotence, associated with other antihypertensive drugs. They do not adversely affect levels of cholesterol, glucose (blood sugar), or uric acid. The most common side effect is an irritating dry cough, which occurs in about 15 percent of people who try ACE inhibitors.

As with diuretics and beta blockers, ACE inhibitors may be less effective in people who take nonsteroidal anti-inflammatory drugs (NSAIDs) such as aspirin or ibuprofen. Taking an antacid with your ACE inhibitor may also prevent all medication from being absorbed in your body. ACE inhibitors can increase the level of potassium dangerously when combined with NSAIDs, potassium supplements, or potassium-sparing diuretics. ACE inhibitors may also increase the amount of lithium in the blood in people taking this drug. Depending on the dose prescribed, ACE inhibitors may need to be taken once or twice a day.

The table on page 130 lists brand and generic names of some commonly prescribed ACE inhibitors. The dosage range given is that recommended by the Joint National Committee on Detection, Evaluation, and Treatment of High Blood Pressure. (Some of these drugs may no longer be available.) Do not change the dose you are taking without talking to your physician.

COMBINATION DRUGS

Combination drugs blend two different blood pressure medications in a single pill or capsule. Various types of combination drugs are now available and more will be developed in the future. By combining the actions of two different drugs, these medications are often more effective for some people than single drugs. In addition, the newer combination drugs use smaller doses of each medication, which reduces the risk of side effects.

One newer low-dose combination drug, which goes by the brand name Ziac, combines the beta blocker bisoprolol fumarate with the diuretic hydrochlorothiazide. Ziac is approved by the

ANGIOTENSIN CONVERTING
ENZYME INHIBITORS

GENERIC NAME	BRAND NAME	ADULT DOSAGE (MILLIGRAMS/DAY)
Benazepril	Lotensin	10 to 40
Captopril	Capoten	12.5 to 150.0
Enalapril	Vasotec	2.5 to 40.0
Fosinopril	Monopril	10 to 40
Lisinopril	Prinivil, Zestril	5 to 40
Quinapril	Accupril	5 to 80
Ramipril	Altace	1.25 to 20.0

USFDA as an initial drug therapy for hypertension. (Other combination drugs are prescribed only for people who have not been able to control their hypertension by taking a single medication.) Ziac, which is taken once a day, is effective in reducing both diastolic and systolic pressure in people who have mild to moderate hypertension. The drug causes few side effects and those that occur are usually mild and temporary. When you first start taking Ziac, you may feel drowsy; in that case, your doctor will recommend avoiding driving a motor vehicle or operating machinery until the drowsiness stops. Because the medication can make your skin more sensitive to the sun, you should always wear a sunscreen with a sun protection factor (SPF) of at least 15 and protective clothing. You should not take the medication if you are allergic to sulfa; call your doctor immediately if you have symptoms of an allergic reaction, including a rash, itching, or difficulty breathing. The effects of Ziac on a developing fetus are not known, so talk to your doctor about switching to another medication if you are pregnant.

Several medications are available that combine an ACE inhibitor and a calcium channel blocker in one pill, including Lexxel, Lotrel, Tarka, and Teczem (brand names). These medications are often prescribed to people who cannot control their blood pressure with a single drug. Lexxel combines enalapril and felodipine and is taken once daily. Side effects are few and mild and include headache, dizziness, and ankle swelling. Lotrel is a combination of amlodipine and benazepril. Tarka includes trandolapril and verapamil. Teczem combines enalapril and diltiazem. The most frequent side effects for any of these combination drugs are headache, dizziness, ankle swelling, and, to a lesser degree, dry cough and constipation. Because all these medications contain an ACE inhibitor, any woman who discovers she is pregnant should talk to her doctor as soon as possible about switching to a different drug.

Another combination drug combines the diuretic hydrochlorothiazide with the angiotensin blocker losartan (brand name, Hyzaar). Possible side effects of this medication include dizziness, weakness, fatigue, muscle cramps, and stomach pain.

Some of the older combination drugs blend an ACE inhibitor with the diuretic hydrochlorothiazide. Brand names include Prinzide, Vaseretic, and Zestoretic. Possible side effects include weakness, dizziness, fatigue, dry cough, headache, and ankle swelling. ACE inhibitor/diuretic combination drugs are recommended mainly for people in whom treatment with diuretics or beta blockers alone was not effective or caused unacceptable side effects. The combination therapy is usually prescribed only after a person has already used the specific ACE inhibitor and diuretic in carefully measured individual doses. If your doctor recommends this therapy, he or she will monitor your blood pressure to make sure it doesn't fall to too low a level, which can sometimes occur when first starting the combination therapy. If you become pregnant while taking the medication, tell your doctor right away. You may need to switch to another therapy.

ALPHA BLOCKERS

Like beta blockers, alpha blockers are adrenergic inhibitors. They have proved effective in controlling blood pressure in all groups of people with hypertension and have been successfully combined with all other types of antihypertensive medication.

While beta blockers interfere with receptors responsive to the hormone norepinephrine in the heart and kidneys, alpha blockers tackle receptors (alpha receptors) in the arteries themselves. By preventing norepinephrine from reaching the receptors, alpha blockers allow the arteries to relax and open wider, thereby lowering blood pressure. One drug in this group, labetalol, combines a beta blocker and an alpha blocker to block all norepinephrine receptors related to blood pressure control. This type of drug is called an alpha-beta blocker.

Because their action on the arteries is so specific and so powerful, the first dose of an alpha blocker may cause a dramatic drop in blood pressure along with fainting or feeling faint. This can be avoided by starting at a very low dose and by taking the medication at night. Using alpha blockers with another antihypertensive drug, especially a diuretic, can cause postural hypotension (abnormally low blood pressure that occurs when a person sits up or stands suddenly), so care must be taken in combination therapy.

Other side effects associated with alpha blockers include rash, headache, dizziness, and mild fluid retention.

Alpha blockers may be particularly useful in people with high blood cholesterol, diabetes, peripheral vascular disease, or an enlarged prostate.

The table below shows dosages recommended by the Joint National Committee on Detection, Evaluation, and Treatment of High Blood Pressure for some commonly prescribed alpha blockers and the alpha-beta blocker labetalol. Do not change doses of your medication without talking to your doctor.

ALPHA AND ALPHA-BETA BLOCKERS

GENERIC NAME	BRAND NAME	ADULT DOSAGE (MILLIGRAMS/DAY)
Doxazosin	Cardura	1 to 16
Labetalol	Normodyne, Trandate	200 to 1,200
Prazosin	Minipress	1 to 20
Terazosin	Hytrin	1 to 20

ANGIOTENSIN BLOCKERS

The first cousins of ACE inhibitors, angiotensin II receptor-blockers, block the ability of angiotensin II to constrict the arteries. Angiotensin blockers also prevent angiotensin II from triggering the kidneys to produce renin and in turn retain salt and water.

Two angiotensin blockers currently available, losartan (brand name, Cozaar) and valsartan (brand name, Diovan), produce a gradual, 24-hour reduction in blood pressure. Losartan is given at doses of 50 to 100 milligrams (usually one 50-milligram pill twice a day if the higher dose is needed). The optimal dose range of valsartan is 80 to 160 mg, one pill per day. Studies that used ambulatory blood pressure monitors showed that losartan maintains a reduced blood pressure that mirrors the normal pattern of blood pressure changes throughout the day and night. Side effects are mild and include dizziness, fatigue, and stomach pain. Angiotensin blockers tend to raise low potassium levels in the blood and to lower high uric acid levels, both of which are useful side effects. People who use these medications generally do not experience postural hypotension (abnormally low blood pressure that occurs when a person sits up or stands suddenly), which may be helpful for older adults. However, these drugs are less effective in blacks and cannot be used by pregnant women.

10

Supplemental Drugs

Because newer antihypertensive medications offer more selective action against high blood pressure and cause fewer side effects, the drugs described in this chapter are now considered supplemental drugs. This means that they are no longer a doctor's first choice for treating hypertension. Although they have been used for many years and are effective at lowering blood pressure, these drugs work by causing very broad effects in the brain, nervous system, or vascular system that make them impractical for general, regular use. Nevertheless, these drugs remain the best choice for some people, and they may be used to treat severe or emergency hypertension because they can be counted on to lower blood pressure.

CENTRALLY ACTING DRUGS

Centrally acting drugs act directly on the brain by altering the central site of blood pressure control. However, this area of the brain and sympathetic nervous system is also responsible for many other functions, including sexual arousal. Like beta blockers and alpha blockers, centrally acting drugs are antiadrenergic, meaning that they target brain cells that release the hormone norepinephrine. More specifically, they lock into receptors that, when occupied by the drug, decrease the activity of the sympathetic nervous system (see Chapter 1). By preventing transmission of these signals, these drugs cause the heart rate to drop and total peripheral resistance to decrease, thereby lowering blood pressure.

People over age 70 in particular may be sensitive to the total effect of these drugs on their central nervous system and should avoid taking them if possible. On the other hand, because these drugs work directly on the nervous system, they are safe for pregnant women and for people with diabetes, kidney disease, or high cholesterol levels. Centrally acting drugs continue to be the best choice for some people.

Centrally acting drugs can cause drowsiness, memory problems, dry mouth, fatigue, and dizziness in some people. Other adverse effects associated with these drugs include postural hypotension (abnormally low blood pressure that occurs when a person sits up or stands suddenly), sexual dysfunction, and decreased mental activity (sharpness). One centrally acting drug, methyldopa, may also cause liver damage, fever, and a low blood count. However, these side effects are uncommon.

A major concern with these drugs, especially clonidine, is their tendency to cause withdrawal symptoms if they are abruptly stopped for any reason. Withdrawal symptoms include headache, nausea, vomiting, and a sharp, sudden rise in blood pressure that may require emergency treatment. Using a skin patch to deliver the medication lessens the possibility of withdrawal symptoms. Fewer side effects have been reported for all centrally acting drugs when people use longer-acting versions.

The table below lists the brand names and generic names of some commonly prescribed centrally acting drugs, along with the dosage recommended by the Joint National Committee on Detection, Evaluation, and Treatment of High Blood Pressure. Do not change doses of any medication you are taking without talking to your physician.

PERIPHERALLY ACTING DRUGS

While centrally acting drugs target cells in the brain, peripherally acting drugs act on nerve cells throughout the body to prevent the release of the hormone norepinephrine. These drugs are not

CENTRALLY ACTING ANTIHYPERTENSIVE DRUGS

GENERIC NAME	BRAND NAME	ADULT DOSAGE (MILLIGRAMS/DAY)
Clonidine	Catapres	0.1 to 1.2
Clonidine (patch)	Catapres-TTS	0.1 to 0.3
Guanabenz	Wytensin	4 to 64
Guanfacine	Tenex	1 to 3
Methyldopa	Aldomet	250 to 2,000

very selective in their action and cause many unpleasant side effects, including diarrhea, postural hypotension (abnormally low blood pressure that occurs when a person sits up or stands suddenly), fatigue, stuffy nose, depression, sexual dysfunction, dry mouth, fluid retention, and increased risk of ulcer. These drugs are not commonly used.

The table below lists the brand names and generic names of some commonly prescribed peripherally acting drugs, along with the dosage recommended by the Joint National Committee on Detection, Evaluation, and Treatment of High Blood Pressure. Do not change doses of any medication you are taking without talking to your physician.

DIRECT VASODILATORS

As their name suggests, direct vasodilators act directly on the smooth muscle in arterial walls, causing the arteries to widen and blood pressure to drop. Because these drugs are so potent, they are generally used only for emergency situations or when a per-

PERIPHERALLY ACTING ANTIHYPERTENSIVE DRUGS

GENERIC NAME	BRAND NAME	ADULT DOSAGE (MILLIGRAMS/DAY)
Guanadrel	Hylorel	10 to 75
Guanethidine	Ismelin	10 to 100
Rauwolfia serpentina	Raudixin	50 to 200
Reserpine	Sandril, Serpasil	0.05 to 0.25

son's blood pressure cannot be adequately controlled by other drugs, alone or in combination.

The side effects caused by direct vasodilators are related to their action and the body's attempt to compensate for the relaxed arteries. People often experience an abnormally strong, rapid heartbeat (usually over 100 beats per minute), increased fluid retention, and headache. Patients with coronary artery disease are at increased risk for having a heart attack, and people taking hydralazine may develop an unpleasant skin condition similar to lupus erythematosus.

Two direct vasodilators, hydralazine (brand name, Apresoline) and minoxidil (brand name, Loniten), can be prescribed for use at home. Depending on how they are used, these drugs are usually taken two or more times per day. Three other direct vasodilators are used only in emergency situations to control blood pressure and are administered intravenously (directly into a vein): diazoxide, nitroglycerin, and sodium nitroprusside.

11

Emergency Situations

A hypertensive emergency occurs when excessively high blood pressure is causing organ damage or may soon cause a heart attack or stroke. If you ever experience a sudden, sharp rise in blood pressure, call your doctor immediately or, if you have symptoms of a hypertensive crisis (see the list on page 141), seek medical help immediately.

What triggers a sudden, dangerous increase in blood pressure (see Chapter 4) is often unknown. It is unusual for a person who is already being treated for high blood pressure to have a hypertensive crisis. In most cases, one health problem causes a chain reaction of events, all of which contribute to the rapid and dangerous rise in blood pressure. Despite the serious symptoms, severely elevated blood pressure is often discovered coincidentally

SYMPTOMS OF A HYPERTENSIVE CRISIS

Warning: If you have symptoms of a hypertensive crisis, call 911 or the emergency medical assistance for your area, or go directly to the nearest hospital emergency department. Symptoms of a hypertensive crisis include the following:

- Headache
- Vomiting
- Dizziness
- Blurred vision (including temporary blindness)
- Chest pain
- Palpitations (an abnormally strong, rapid heartbeat)
- Shortness of breath
- Seizures
- Stupor (decreased responsiveness)
- Coma

when a doctor is examining a patient for some other health problem. The average age of people who experience a hypertensive crisis is 40, and men are affected more often than women.

WHAT IS A HYPERTENSIVE EMERGENCY?

Because a hypertensive emergency requires that blood pressure be reduced within the hour to prevent or limit organ damage, it is critical to identify such emergencies quickly and accurately. But lowering a person's blood pressure too rapidly can cause other serious health problems (for example, the brain could be deprived of oxygen because of decreased blood flow). Because of these risks, it is vital to determine the extent of the emergency before beginning treatment.

No definite guidelines outline precisely what constitutes a hypertensive emergency. Blood pressure alone is not the defining factor. The person's age, health history (including how long he or she has had hypertension), kidney function, duration of hypertension, and speed of onset of blood pressure elevation are all important factors in determining whether there is an emergency. Rapid onset of severely elevated blood pressure in a young, previously healthy person would cause more concern than it would in an older person who is known to have hypertension.

Doctors usually treat the following conditions as hypertensive emergencies:

- Aortic dissection (a tear in the largest artery in the body)
- Acute left ventricular failure and pulmonary edema (fluid in the lungs)
- Acute kidney failure or worsening of chronic kidney failure
- Preeclampsia and eclampsia (see Chapter 12)
- Hypertensive encephalopathy (a disease of the brain)
- Stroke (caused by a blocked or torn artery)
- Pheochromocytoma (see Chapter 2)
- Cocaine overdose
- Unstable angina or heart attack

EVALUATING A HYPERTENSIVE CRISIS

When a person's systolic blood pressure (the first of the two numbers in a blood pressure reading) is 200 mm Hg or higher and/or the diastolic blood pressure (the second of the two numbers) is over 120 mm Hg, the doctor will check the blood pressure in the person's other arm. Blood pressure should be measured again in both arms 10 minutes later. Measuring blood pressure while the person is in different positions (that is, sitting, standing, and lying down) may also be helpful. If the person is a pregnant woman, the doctor will contact her obstetrician immediately.

Then the doctor needs to determine whether brain function has been affected. This helps him or her to establish whether a stroke has occurred or if there is other brain damage. Symptoms of possible brain damage include headache, dizziness, and lethargy. A headache alone with very high blood pressure is usually not a hypertensive emergency. Checking the arteries in the back of the eyes will tell the doctor whether these or other blood vessels have been damaged by the severe hypertension. The combination of severe hypertension and papilledema (swelling of the optic nerve) often prompts the doctor to treat the situation aggressively as a hypertensive emergency.

After the doctor has checked brain function, he or she must determine the condition of the heart. The doctor will check for enlargement of the heart, heart failure (demonstrated by fluid in the lungs), and differences in pulse rate in the arms and legs. If the doctor is concerned about a possible heart attack or other heart disorders, the person will need to have an electrocardiogram (ECG, a test of the electrical activity of the heart muscle), a chest X ray, and blood tests. These blood tests, along with a urinalysis, will provide information on kidney function.

The doctor will also need to know about drug use, including prescription drugs (especially whether the person may have recently skipped a dose of medication for hypertension, heart disease, or kidney disease) and illegal recreational drugs (especially cocaine and amphetamines). Combinations of certain drugs can cause interactions that lead to a sudden, dangerous rise in blood pressure.

TREATING A HYPERTENSIVE EMERGENCY

The goal in treating a hypertensive emergency is the prompt but gradual reduction of blood pressure to a reasonable (but still hypertensive) level. This usually means bringing blood pressure down to 150 to 160/100 to 110 mm Hg within several hours and maintaining it at this level for a few days. Lowering blood pressure too quickly or too much can impair the body's ability to regulate blood flow. This can result in too little blood (and oxygen) reaching the heart, brain, kidneys, and other organs. Once blood pressure has been stabilized, additional antihypertensive treatment can be started or resumed.

Hypertensive emergencies must be treated with medication given intravenously (through a needle inserted into a vein). Medication delivered directly into the bloodstream produces the quickest response, and the doctor can control how much medication is injected, thus lowering blood pressure gradually. In some cases, however, medication placed under the tongue or taken by mouth may be used to quickly and safely manage a hypertensive emergency. The doctor will choose an appropriate drug based on the person's symptoms, identified organ damage, and other health factors, such as a possible stroke. Many of the drugs used in emergency treatment of hypertension must be used carefully.

Understandably, some people may panic when they see that their blood pressure is so high. However, if you or a loved one experience a dramatic increase in blood pressure but have no other symptoms, do not be surprised if the doctor provides treatment in the office. Only genuine medical emergencies need to be treated as such, and the doctor will determine when the situation warrants hospitalization and emergency treatment.

12

Hypertension During Pregnancy

More than 10 percent of all pregnant women develop high blood pressure. Blood pressure monitoring is critical throughout pregnancy because hypertension can harm both the woman and her fetus. If high blood pressure develops during pregnancy in a woman who previously had normal blood pressure, the condition is called preeclampsia (or toxemia of pregnancy). However, women who are mildly to moderately hypertensive (but whose blood pressure is controlled with medication) before becoming pregnant usually face no additional risks unless they also have kidney disease. Pregnant women who take blood pressure medication may need to change the type or dose of medication.

Systolic blood pressure does not change much during pregnancy. Normally, diastolic blood pressure goes down 5 to 10 mm Hg during pregnancy, reaching its lowest point in the middle trimester of the pregnancy. Blood pressure then gradually returns to about the prepregnancy level just before delivery. The reason for this drop in blood pressure is that the hormone progesterone causes blood vessels to dilate (widen) at this point in the pregnancy.

PREEXISTING HYPERTENSION

Because many women do not plan their pregnancies, women with hypertension may conceive while taking medication. For this reason, most doctors prescribe drugs that are safe to take during pregnancy for women of childbearing age with hypertension. If you become pregnant, do not stop taking your blood pressure medication; doing so may cause a sudden or sharp increase in blood pressure and put you and your fetus at risk. Let your doctor know that your are pregnant; he or she will recommend any changes that might be required to manage your blood pressure. Two main objectives govern the treatment of hypertension during pregnancy: controlling the woman's blood pressure and allowing the fetus to grow and develop normally.

Many blood pressure medications are safe to take during pregnancy, and doctors often recommend continuing the same drug if it was working well before the pregnancy. Diuretics are seldom recommended during pregnancy because they can reduce blood volume. For women taking the beta blocker propranolol, doctors may suggest switching to another drug in the same class, because propranolol can affect uterine blood flow early in pregnancy.

Warning: Angiotensin converting enzyme (ACE) inhibitors must be avoided because they can cause serious problems to the fetus, including death.

CHANGES IN BLOOD PRESSURE DURING PREGNANCY

Some change in blood pressure is expected during pregnancy. Women are not diagnosed as hypertensive unless their systolic blood pressure increases 30 mm Hg or more or their diastolic blood pressure increases 15 mm Hg or more. If a woman's baseline blood pressure before becoming pregnant is not known, any reading of 140/90 mm Hg or higher is considered abnormal.

The timing of the elevation in blood pressure also affects the diagnosis and treatment. If hypertension is discovered before the 20th week of pregnancy, the woman is treated as though she had preexisting hypertension. It simply may be that her hypertension had not been diagnosed or that high blood pressure was in the process of developing when she became pregnant. In this case, the woman is treated as described in the previous section (Preexisting Hypertension). However, some women with preexisting hypertension develop preeclampsia. Doctors diagnose preeclampsia in a woman who already has hypertension by monitoring her blood pressure, the amount of protein in her urine, and the amount of swelling she experiences.

High blood pressure diagnosed after the 20th week of pregnancy may be classified as preeclampsia, eclampsia, or transient hypertension, depending on the other symptoms and circumstances. Whether mild or severe, however, preeclampsia is serious. The condition is caused by constriction (narrowing) of the blood vessels, which reduces the blood supply to tissues, including the fetus and placenta (the organ that develops in the uterus during pregnancy, connecting the blood supplies of the woman and fetus). Women with preeclampsia have elevated blood pressure, proteinuria (protein in the urine), and edema (swelling) that is most noticeable in the hands and face. The reduced blood flow to the placenta threatens the health and development of the fetus. Preeclampsia may also cause kidney damage in the woman.

Women planning to become pregnant can take steps to reduce their risk of developing preeclampsia. Research shows that women who take 1,500 to 2,000 milligrams of calcium in supplements daily are only one third as likely to develop preeclampsia as women who do not take the supplements. Taking calcium supplements also may reduce the risk of premature birth and fetal growth retardation. Some foods are also a good source of calcium (see table on page 150).

Preeclampsia usually occurs during a first pregnancy. Women who are young, have diabetes, are carrying twins, or have a previous history of high blood pressure are at increased risk for preeclampsia. Some research suggests that women who are resistant to the effects of insulin (see Chapter 14) are also more likely to develop preeclampsia.

Mild preeclampsia is diagnosed when two blood pressure readings taken at least 6 hours apart show an increase in systolic blood pressure (upper reading) of at least 30 mm Hg or an increase in diastolic blood pressure (lower reading) of at least 15 mm Hg, and when 0.3 gram (0.01 ounces) or more of protein are present in the urine over a 24-hour period. The fluid retention that accompanies this condition usually occurs as swelling or rapid weight gain.

Preeclampsia is defined as severe when any of the following signs or symptoms occur after the 20th week of pregnancy:

- Systolic blood pressure above 160 mm Hg
- Diastolic blood pressure above 110 mm Hg
- Presence of 5.0 grams or more of protein in the urine in a 24-hour period
- Reduction in the amount of urine normally produced (500 milliliters or less in 24 hours)
- Blurred vision
- Fluid in the lungs
- Cyanosis (bluish or purplish skin color)
- Pain in the upper abdomen

Doctors treating preeclampsia want to slow the progression of the disease, both to protect the woman and to allow the fetus to develop in the uterus for as long as possible. They usually first recommend bed rest at home to prevent blood pressure from rising any further. A lying position allows greater blood flow to the uterus, which lowers blood pressure and improves circulation to the fetus. In mild cases, a few hours of rest throughout the day may be sufficient. In severe cases, complete bed rest, possibly in the hospital, may be required.

Women with preeclampsia are encouraged to get more calcium, either through their diet (see table on page 150) or supplements. All pregnant women should stop drinking alcohol and smoking at the start of pregnancy. For women with preeclampsia, these habits are especially dangerous—both alcohol consumption and cigarette smoking raise blood pressure and can directly harm the fetus.

In cases of severe preeclampsia in which the pregnancy is be-

GOOD SOURCES OF CALCIUM

FOOD	SERVING SIZE	CALCIUM (MILLIGRAMS)
1% low-fat milk	1 cup	350
Calcium-fortified orange juice	1 cup	320
Low-fat yogurt	1 cup	300
Collard greens, cooked	½ cup	180
Salmon, canned (with bones)	3 ounces	170
Spinach, cooked	½ cup	140
Calcium-fortified tofu	4 ounces	150
Low-fat cottage cheese	1 cup	120
Corn tortilla	2	120
Great northern beans	½ cup	105
Kale, cooked	½ cup	100

yond 30 weeks, delivery of the baby is usually thought to be the best course, to protect the woman from stroke and other life-threatening complications. Antihypertensive drugs are usually used, but with caution, at this time.

One rare type of preeclampsia includes small variations in blood pressure, a slight drop in blood platelet count, and mild elevations in liver enzymes. While this combination of symptoms is not necessarily dangerous, it can progress quickly to a life-threatening condition known as HELLP (hemolysis, elevated liver enzymes, low platelet count) syndrome. Women diagnosed with HELLP syndrome must either deliver or have the pregnancy ended, depending on the stage of pregnancy.

In any case of preeclampsia, it is sometimes necessary to deliver the fetus as an emergency measure before the pregnancy is complete. An emergency delivery is performed whenever there are signs of prolonged fetal distress, uncontrollable hypertension in the woman, kidney or liver failure in the woman, upper abdominal pain, or signs of impending eclampsia. If delivery is imminent and the woman's condition worsens, antihypertensive drugs may be administered intravenously (directly into a vein).

Women with either mild or severe preeclampsia are always at risk of developing eclampsia—a much more serious condition that poses a danger to both woman (seizures, organ damage, death) and fetus (premature delivery, death). Headache, stomach pain, blurred vision, and facial twitching usually precede the seizures, but occasionally eclampsia may develop without warning.

Not all pregnant women who develop high blood pressure experience these serious complications. Some women experience a rise in blood pressure with no other symptoms during pregnancy or within 24 hours of delivery. This condition is called transient hypertension. In this case, a woman should have her blood pressure monitored after the child is born.

OTHER BLOOD PRESSURE CONCERNS FOR WOMEN

Taking birth control pills is linked with high blood pressure in some women. You should have your blood pressure checked before starting the pill, 2 to 3 months later, and then yearly thereafter. Your blood pressure is more likely to rise if you are overweight, have had hypertension during pregnancy, or have kidney disease or a family history of high blood pressure. As discussed in Chapter 2, being overweight or gaining weight increases the possibility of developing high blood pressure regardless of whether you use birth control pills. The combination of birth control pills and cigarette smoking can be especially dangerous, particularly for women over age 35. If your blood pressure rises when you use birth control pills, your doctor will probably adjust the dose or recommend switching to a different form of contraception. Your blood pressure should return to normal levels within a few months of stopping the pill.

Before menopause, most women are at little risk of developing coronary heart disease. Unless their hypertension is severe, younger women should generally first try to make lifestyle changes (see Chapter 6) to lower their blood pressure before turning to blood pressure medication. After menopause, when the ovaries stop producing estrogen, women are at greater risk of developing hypertension than are men. A woman's risk of heart disease of any sort goes up after menopause. Some women who use estrogen replacement therapy may experience a slight rise in their blood pressure. All postmenopausal women should regularly monitor their blood pressure regardless of whether they are taking estrogen.

Black women, even young black women, are much more susceptible to high blood pressure than are white women. Hypertension in black women tends to be more serious as well. Among women over 65, one survey showed that 83 percent of black women have hypertension, compared with 66 percent of white women. Treatment of hypertension in black women must take into account the unique blood pressure profile found in most blacks (see Chapter 13).

13

Hypertension in Special Groups

Doctors have long recognized that hypertension is particularly common in certain groups of people, such as African Americans and older adults. These and other groups, such as children, require special consideration when evaluating hypertension and planning treatment. Information that applies to these groups has been provided throughout this book. This chapter summarizes some important characteristics of high blood pressure as it relates to African Americans, older adults, and children.

AFRICAN AMERICANS

High blood pressure is twice as common in blacks as it is in whites. The disease tends to develop earlier in life in African

Americans and is usually more severe. Secondary (and thus curable) hypertension is less common in blacks than in whites. Both blacks and whites from the southeastern US have a greater risk of and higher death rates from stroke than other regions of the country. Studies showed that 11 states have stroke death rates that are 10 percent or more above the national average. These states, including Alabama, Arkansas, Georgia, Indiana, Kentucky, Louisiana, Mississippi, North Carolina, South Carolina, Tennessee, and Virginia, are sometimes referred to as the "stroke belt." Although the degree to which heredity versus environment plays a role has not yet been determined, hypertension does tend to run in African American families and is most common in black women.

In a study of older African Americans with hypertension and chronic kidney problems, those who said they were less satisfied with their medical care were also less likely to follow medication instructions and were more likely to report symptoms related to antihypertensive drug use. It is important for people with hypertension to take an active role in their treatment planning and blood pressure management to ensure satisfaction with treatment and outcome.

As a group, African Americans have hypertension characterized by low renin activity (see Chapter 1) and increased peripheral resistance (the degree to which blood vessels resist blood flow). African Americans are more likely to have organ damage related to their hypertension, such as stroke, left ventricular hypertrophy, and kidney disease. Hypertension combined with diabetes or insulin resistance syndrome (see Chapter 14) accounts for much of the end-stage kidney disease seen in African Americans.

African Americans are likely to be salt sensitive and their hypertension is likely to respond both to weight loss and salt restriction. Their hypertension responds well to diuretics also, but they are likely to require a second medication (both at low dose), such as an angiotensin converting enzyme (ACE) inhibitor. Calcium channel blockers, beta blockers, alpha blockers, and alpha-beta blockers are all equally effective in blacks and whites.

More helpful information about the treatment of high blood pressure in blacks will come out of the African American Study of Kidney Disease and Hypertension (AASK), which is described in more detail in Chapter 15.

OLDER ADULTS

Although blood pressure tends to increase with age, this change is not inevitable, particularly among people who live low-stress, active lives. Doctors must be especially careful in monitoring blood pressure in their older patients. In one study of repeated blood pressure measurements (one reading after another over a 20-minute period), blood pressure in older people dropped with each successive reading. The researchers suggested that allowing older people to relax for 15 minutes before a blood pressure check may result in a more accurate reading.

In many older adults, only systolic blood pressure goes up. Throughout the body, arteries become stiffer and lose their elasticity over the years. The main artery in the body, the aorta, experiences the same changes and cannot expand as much when the heart pumps blood through it. Because the aorta is stiff, the heart has to pump harder, and systolic blood pressure is elevated. This is called isolated systolic hypertension.

Recent clinical studies have shown that treating hypertension is quite beneficial for older adults, perhaps even more so than for younger adults. A study in Europe found that treatment to lower blood pressure resulted in fewer strokes and heart attacks in older adults with isolated systolic hypertension. An analysis of all studies of hypertension treatment in older adults—even those with mild to moderate hypertension—noted that treatment lowered the risk of death, stroke, heart attack, congestive heart failure, and other related health problems. However, in patients above age 85, most doctors do not recommend starting new treatment for mildly elevated blood pressure; stopping existing treatment is not recommended either.

Because older people are particularly sensitive to medication, antihypertensive drugs should be prescribed with caution at a dose lower than the normally recommended starting level. Dose adjustments should be made slowly at 6- to 8-week intervals. Older adults are more prone to postural hypotension (abnormally low blood pressure that occurs when a person suddenly stands or sits up), so blood pressure should be checked in standing, sitting, and lying positions. This will indicate whether the medication is causing excessively low blood pressure following changes in position. Drugs likely to cause postural hypotension should be avoided.

CHILDREN

Hypertension is rare among children. However, the lifestyle habits a child learns while growing up can affect his or her blood pressure and can increase the chances of developing hypertension in adulthood. Poor diet, little activity, weight gain, and smoking in childhood all increase the likelihood of adult hypertension. In addition, children whose parents have hypertension are 20 percent to 30 percent more likely to develop high blood pressure than children whose parents have normal blood pressure levels.

The pediatrician should measure your child's blood pressure during routine health examinations starting as early as when the child is 3 years old. A child with a slight elevation may need monitoring and another blood pressure check within 3 to 6 months, while a child with significantly elevated blood pressure should be checked again within a few days to a week. Children with early signs of essential hypertension usually have only mildly elevated blood pressure.

Hypertension in children is diagnosed according to the results of three or more separate blood pressure readings. Appropriate cuff size is very important in measuring blood pressure in children, and special blood pressure monitors are required for infants. Blood pressure readings in the upper ranges usually indicate secondary hypertension. Children who have blood pressure that is high-normal or significantly elevated on occasion should be monitored regularly for hypertension and other risk factors for heart disease, such as high blood cholesterol levels. Children who have been diagnosed with type I diabetes are likely to develop hypertension also, often as a result of kidney damage.

The probable causes of hypertension in children change with age. Among infants and young children, kidney disease, coarctation of the aorta (a defect present from birth), and blockage of the renal artery (the artery that supplies blood to the kidney) are most likely to raise blood pressure. In school-age children, both sec-

CLASSIFICATION OF HYPERTENSION IN CHILDREN BY AGE

AGE GROUP	HIGH-NORMAL*		SIGNIFICANT HYPERTENSION*		SEVERE HYPERTENSION*	
	SYSTOLIC	DIASTOLIC	SYSTOLIC	DIASTOLIC	SYSTOLIC	DIASTOLIC
7 days	—	—	96 to 105	—	≥ 106	—
8 to 30 days	—	—	104 to 109	—	≥ 110	—
≤ 2 years	104 to 111	70 to 73	112 to 117	74 to 81	≥ 118	≥ 82
3 to 5 years	108 to 115	70 to 75	116 to 123	76 to 83	≥ 124	≥ 84
6 to 9 years	114 to 121	74 to 77	122 to 129	78 to 85	≥ 130	≥ 86
10 to 12 years	122 to 125	78 to 81	126 to 133	82 to 89	≥ 134	≥ 90
13 to 15 years	130 to 135	80 to 85	136 to 143	86 to 89	≥ 144	≥ 92
16 to 18 years	136 to 141	84 to 91	142 to 149	92 to 97	≥ 150	≥ 98

*Measurements are in mm Hg.
Key: $\leq$ means less than or equal to; $\geq$ means greater than or equal to.

ondary (due mainly to kidney disorders) and essential hypertension occur. In adolescents, essential hypertension is most common, followed by secondary hypertension caused by kidney disease. Use of alcohol, cigarettes, cocaine, or other addictive substances may also cause increased blood pressure in children and adolescents, as can steroid use. Neurofibromatosis, Turner's syndrome, heart failure, and other disorders can also cause secondary hypertension in children.

As in adults, body weight and weight gain are directly related to blood pressure in children. Efforts to prevent childhood obesity may be useful in preventing adult hypertension and adult obesity. Low physical fitness and activity levels are generally linked with higher levels of body fat. Not surprisingly, then, in elementary school children, systolic blood pressure has been found to be highest in children with poor physical fitness. Children with uncomplicated hypertension should be encouraged to exercise regularly.

Although stroke, heart attack, kidney failure, and other complications of high blood pressure seem a long way off, you must realize that hypertension in an otherwise healthy, active child is not a harmless condition. Treatment planning must be individualized. Because the long-term effects of antihypertensive drugs on children who are growing and developing are largely unknown, and because it is likely that treatment for hypertension will be lifelong, the issue about whether to give blood pressure medication to children is a matter of serious debate. Except in cases of curable secondary hypertension, treatment usually focuses on supporting lifestyle changes and heart-healthy habits.

This is particularly true regarding diet. Researchers now believe that what people eat during adolescence and young adulthood greatly affects future health. Children establish their food preferences early and learn from example. Therefore, eating a healthy, balanced diet must be a family activity. If your child has or is at risk for high blood pressure, gradually reduce the amount of fat and salt in his or her diet. Children over the age of 2 years who are at risk for hypertension or heart disease can safely drink nonfat milk and should be encouraged to eat low-fat dairy products. Fresh fruits and vegetables and whole-grain products should also be standard fare in the household. If your child needs to lose weight, avoid emphasizing favorite but forbidden foods to help prevent development of a possible eating disorder. Instead, as described in Chapter 6, make meaningful, permanent changes in eating patterns that will last a lifetime and promote a healthy body weight.

Exercise and general physical activity are important both to help maintain a healthy body weight and to strengthen your child's cardiovascular system. Daily walking, bicycling, and other outdoor play should be encouraged. If safety is a concern, find a supervised, age-appropriate sport or group activity for your child to join. Be sure to tell your school and parents' groups that you support regular and after-school physical education programs. At home, you may need to limit the total amount of time spent watching television, using a computer, or playing video games to ensure that your child remains physically active.

14

Hypertension and Other Disease

Because hypertension increases your risk of developing other diseases, your doctor will watch closely for signs of new health problems. Often, people with hypertension also have other disorders, such as diabetes, insulin resistance, or atherosclerosis. Whenever a person has two or more health problems at the same time, the doctor must ensure that treatment of one disease does not interfere with treatment of another. This is particularly important with regard to medications. This chapter reviews medical conditions that often occur along with hypertension and that may require special monitoring and treatment.

DIABETES

Diabetes is the inability of the body to maintain normal blood sugar levels. There are two types of diabetes. Type I (insulin-dependent) diabetes usually starts in childhood or young adulthood and accounts for just 5 percent to 10 percent of all cases. People with type I diabetes must inject themselves with insulin to maintain acceptable levels of glucose in their blood. Type II (non–insulin-dependent) diabetes usually occurs around middle age or later and is much more common than type I. People with type II diabetes are generally overweight and often have a history of mild to moderate hypertension. Type II diabetes is managed with diet and exercise. If this treatment is not effective, the doctor may prescribe hypoglycemic medication. Some people may need to take insulin injections to control their blood sugar levels. Just as weight loss usually decreases the effects of hypertension, so it usually lessens the symptoms of type II diabetes. In some cases, type II diabetes may even subside.

An estimated 3 million Americans have both diabetes and hypertension. Hypertension is twice as common in people with diabetes as in the general population. Hypertension tends to occur at the same time that kidney damage is diagnosed in people with type I diabetes. People with type II diabetes often learn about their high blood pressure when their diabetes is diagnosed. African Americans are two times more likely and Mexican Americans are three times more likely to have both hypertension and diabetes than are non-Hispanic whites. In most people with diabetes, hypertension results from increased peripheral resistance (see Chapter 1 for a review of this concept). People with diabetes are also more likely to have isolated systolic hypertension (see Chapter 4).

People with diabetes and hypertension have a greater risk of developing cardiovascular disease, coronary artery disease, and kidney disease than do those with diabetes alone. Both disorders raise the risk of stroke; diabetes increases the risk of stroke by two to four times, and hypertension increases it by six times the average risk. People with diabetes also have a higher level of lipids (fat) in their blood. In addition, both small and large blood vessels thicken abnormally, conditions known as microangiopathy and macroangiopathy, respectively. Diabetes is the leading cause of end-stage kidney disease in the US, and hypertension accelerates the rate of decline in kidney function.

The treatment goal for people with hypertension and diabetes is more rigorous than for people with high blood pressure alone. Your target blood pressure should be 130/85 mm Hg, because of the increased risk for heart disease and related health problems. Blood pressure in people with diabetes fluctuates more over a 24-hour period than it does in people without diabetes, so you may want to monitor your pressure and your glucose levels regularly, even daily, until both are under control.

Weight loss, regular exercise, and avoidance of alcohol and tobacco will improve your ability to maintain satisfactory glucose levels and control your blood pressure. The importance of these lifestyle changes cannot be overstated for anyone with hypertension, and especially for someone who also has diabetes. In people who have stage 1 hypertension and diabetes, a 3-month period of lifestyle modification should be completed before any decision is made about whether antihypertensive medication is needed. If your blood pressure is above 160/100 mm Hg, though, you will probably need to start taking drugs right away. Once your blood pressure is under control, you may be able to rely on lifestyle changes alone.

If drugs are needed to control your blood pressure, care must be taken with almost any medication selected. An angiotensin converting enzyme (ACE) inhibitor should be among the first medications considered, especially when the person has type I diabetes. The doctor must watch for elevated potassium levels and declining kidney function when both renal arteries show evidence of atherosclerosis (a condition more common in people with diabetes). Raised potassium levels can reduce the body's ability to handle glucose.

Calcium channel blockers do not seem to pose problems with regard to glucose control, cholesterol levels, kidney function, or potassium levels. However, these drugs can aggravate postural hypotension (abnormally low blood pressure that occurs when a person sits up or stands suddenly) in people with diabetes. Alpha blockers are also reasonable choices and are often favored because they have positive effects on blood cholesterol levels. However, they, too, can aggravate postural hypotension.

Diuretics, especially potassium-sparing diuretics, will control blood pressure but, like ACE inhibitors, increase the risk of hyperkalemia (high potassium levels in the blood). However, diuretics are often the first choice for treating isolated systolic hypertension. Beta blockers can mask symptoms of hypoglycemia (low blood sugar) and prolong recovery from this state. They also reduce peripheral blood flow, which is already a problem for many people who have diabetes, and they have negative effects on glucose and lipid control.

INSULIN RESISTANCE SYNDROME

Four major risk factors for heart disease often coexist in the same person: obesity, hypertension, high triglyceride levels, and high insulin levels. This "deadly quartet" of risk factors has been called insulin resistance syndrome, or sometimes Reaven's syndrome, after the researcher who first noted the combination of risk factors. Some people with this syndrome also have type II diabetes, and many have an apple-shaped body, with extra fat around their waist. High levels of uric acid and low levels of high density lipoprotein (HDL, or "good") cholesterol in the blood are also common.

The central component in this syndrome is insulin, a hormone produced by the pancreas. Insulin has several functions throughout the body. Insulin triggers certain tissues—skeletal muscle, liver tissue, and adipose (fat) tissue—to remove glucose (sugar) from the blood. After a meal, for example, the glucose level in the blood goes up, and so does the level of insulin. Once enough glucose has been taken out of the blood, the pancreas stops sending out insulin. Insulin also prompts appropriate tissues to make protein and to store fat.

In some people, the skeletal muscles begin to resist the effects of insulin and no longer do their share of removing glucose from the blood. Some researchers believe that lack of exercise causes a change in the muscle cells, lessening their ability to respond to insulin. Whatever the cause, the pancreas must produce more and more insulin to lower blood sugar levels. The excess insulin can increase blood pressure by causing the kidneys to retain salt or by stimulating the sympathetic nervous system (see Chapter 1). Eventually, the liver responds to elevated insulin levels by converting glucose in the blood into triglycerides, which are, in turn, stored as body fat.

Results from the Framingham Heart Study show that for every 10 percent increase in body weight, systolic blood pressure rises 6.5 mm Hg, cholesterol level rises 12 milligrams per deciliter, and fasting blood glucose rises 2 milligrams per deciliter. (An increased fasting glucose level shows that insulin is not doing its job.) Excess body fat is associated with an overproduction of cholesterol by the liver—an increase of 22 milligrams of cholesterol per day for every extra 2 pounds of body weight.

Insulin resistance syndrome can be successfully treated with a combination of regular exercise and a low-fat, low-salt diet (along with the elimination of alcohol, caffeine, and nicotine). Weight loss is essential. A few studies suggest that alpha blockers and ACE inhibitors reduce insulin resistance, so if antihypertensive drug therapy is needed, these medications may be considered first.

VASCULAR DISEASE

Vascular disease refers to problems in the arteries, veins, and other blood vessels throughout the body. In the brain, it is called cerebrovascular disease; in the kidneys, renovascular disease; and in the heart, coronary artery disease. Several vascular disorders that can occur throughout the body are known as peripheral vascular disease. These include blockage of the carotid arteries (large arteries in the neck that supply blood to the head), aneurysms (thin-walled "balloons" or bulges in the arteries), and intermittent claudication (narrowing of arteries supplying muscles in the legs, causing pain upon walking). Hypertension is a risk factor for all of these disorders, and control of blood pressure is an important part of treatment.

Perhaps the most serious type of vascular disease for people with hypertension is coronary artery disease (see Chapter 3). People with diabetes experience atherosclerosis sooner and to a greater extent than most other people. Coronary artery disease is the most common cause of death among people being treated for hypertension. Doctors recognize several risk factors for atherosclerosis (see list below) and watch for them in their patients.

Hypertension in people who also have coronary artery disease is an extremely serious matter. Weight loss, exercise, a low-fat diet, and smoking cessation are generally the best treatment choices in this situation. However, when the risk of heart attack or stroke is high (for example, if the person has hypertension, elevated low density lipoprotein [LDL, or "bad"] cholesterol, and is obese), the doctor will usually combine lifestyle changes with drug treatment. This approach quickly reduces the chances of developing serious complications. Blood pressure should be reduced, as needed, with beta blockers, calcium channel blockers, or combination therapy.

RISK FACTORS FOR ATHEROSCLEROSIS

- Hypertension
- High levels of low density lipoprotein (LDL, or "bad") cholesterol
- Low levels of high density lipoprotein (HDL, or "good") cholesterol
- Cigarette smoking
- Diabetes
- Obesity
- Male
- Family history of premature atherosclerosis

LEFT VENTRICULAR HYPERTROPHY

As you learned in Chapter 3, with hypertension the heart often must work harder to pump blood, and as a result, the heart muscle thickens and becomes less flexible. This can lead to left ventricular hypertrophy, which reduces the ability of the heart to pump blood out to the body tissues. People with left ventricular hypertrophy are at risk for heart attack and heart failure.

Weight loss and salt restriction are often important when the left ventricle is enlarged. Beta blockers, calcium channel blockers, and ACE inhibitors, alone or in low-dose combination therapy, help both the elevated blood pressure and the hypertrophy. Beta blockers also slow the heart rate, allowing more time for the ventricle to fill.

KIDNEY FAILURE

The kidneys are essential in the control of blood pressure (see Chapter 1) and are susceptible to damage caused by elevated blood pressure (see Chapter 3). People with hypertension and kidney failure usually have a common problem: fluid and sodium retention. High doses of diuretics may be required to control both the hypertension and the fluid retention. ACE inhibitors are also beneficial in kidney disease because they help reduce the amount of protein removed in the urine and slow the progression of kidney disease. However, the doctor must monitor levels of potassium and creatinine (a waste product filtered by the kidneys) in the blood to be sure that the drug does not cause additional problems. People with hypertension and kidney failure will also be instructed to make changes in their diet, such as eating less protein and sodium. No matter how the doctor approaches treatment, the goals in kidney failure combined with hypertension are—as in diabetes combined with hypertension—more rigorous than for people with hypertension alone. To protect the kidneys, blood pressure should be reduced to 130/85 mm Hg.

RESPIRATORY DISEASE

Although hypertension is not usually linked to respiratory disease, drug treatment for both conditions can conflict if not managed properly. In people with asthma, bronchitis, or emphysema, beta blockers and alpha-beta blockers can cause the air passages in the lungs to constrict even further and therefore should never be used to control blood pressure in such cases. A dry, unproductive cough, which is a common side effect of ACE inhibitors, can also complicate these respiratory conditions. People with asthma, bronchitis, or emphysema should avoid these drugs.

15

Hypertension Research

The information presented in this book represents the best
available medical advice on the treatment of high blood pressure. Even as you read this, though, researchers are looking for
better ways to diagnose and treat hypertension. The American
Medical Association (AMA) helps researchers share their find-
ings with other doctors and scientists through its medical journals, such as the *Journal of the American Medical Association*
(JAMA) and the *Archives of Internal Medicine.* You probably hear
media reports on medical studies published in *JAMA* and other
journals. However, even when a study has been well conducted
and the results are important to the medical community, you
should never make any treatment decisions based on published
reports of a single clinical study. The study may be very small,

and the results may not apply to someone with your health history. This chapter will help you understand medical research in general and ongoing studies of hypertension in particular. Also, ask your doctor when you have any questions about how a new study might apply to you.

WHAT IS A CLINICAL TRIAL?

You probably decide, on the basis of what you hear from other people and from your doctor, whether a particular medical treatment is effective. But how do doctors determine which treatment works best in which patient? New drugs must first be tested on animals and then on people to determine if they are safe and effective. Then they must be compared with existing drugs to see if the new drugs are any better at treating a particular disease. Medical researchers evaluate any new treatment through a process known as a randomized, controlled, clinical trial.

A clinical trial is any medical study conducted on humans rather than animals. The people who participate in the study may be patients with a specific disease, or they may be healthy volunteers.

A randomized trial is one in which participants in the study are randomly (in no particular order) divided into two or more groups. The groups are divided equally in terms of number and characteristics of participants. In other words, each group must contain equal numbers of men and women, younger people and older people, blacks and whites, and so on. The researchers use a computer to assign study participants to each group.

In a controlled trial, the researchers include one group of participants who receive no treatment at all. If one or more drugs are being studied, the control group will receive what is known as a placebo—an inactive pill or a sugar pill, as it is often called. These individuals know there is a possiblity they are taking a placebo, but none of the study participants knows for sure what is in his or her medication. Including a placebo group (a control group) is especially useful when monitoring the side effects of drugs. In theory, participants taking the placebo should report no side effects. The researchers can then compare the number and types of side effects reported by participants taking the placebo (but who may think they are taking a real, active drug) with those of participants taking active medications. This helps the researchers to identify which side effects are actually caused by the medication being studied.

In some cases, a participant's condition sometimes improves because he or she strongly believes that the treatment will work. This is known as the placebo effect. In clinical trials, researchers compare the improvements in blood pressure of participants taking the placebo with those of participants taking active drugs. This helps them determine whether the chemical in the drug is lowering blood pressure, or whether participants' belief in the drug is causing the improvement.

Some people may feel that every participant should receive the active drug. However, without this type of testing, doctors cannot determine which drugs work the best. If all of the participants in a clinical trial knew which drug they were taking, they might be more likely to say what they thought the researchers wanted to hear. They would also be more likely to believe the drug was working (again, the placebo effect).

A blind trial is another way of ensuring that the true effects of the drug are observed. In a single-blind trial, the researchers know which participants are receiving which pills, but the participants do not. In a double-blind trial, neither the researchers nor the participants know who is taking which pill until the study ends. Double-blind studies are the best type of clinical trial. Because the researchers conducting the study do not know who is taking the real drug, they are less likely to (unintentionally) treat them differently, thereby affecting their perception of the drug.

Large drug studies are often "open label," meaning that both the researchers and the participants know who is taking which drug. This is often easier in very large clinical trials that are comparing well-established treatments. No control group is included in this type of clinical trial.

Finally, the size and duration of a clinical trial varies depending on the type of questions being asked. Smaller studies are used to detect the precise effects of a drug on the body. Participants in these small studies usually undergo many tests. These studies may last a single day or a few weeks. Sometimes the participants must live at the research facility so that the researchers know exactly what they eat, drink, and do while being studied.

Many participants and a longer time span are needed when comparing different treatment methods, or when identifying side effects of one or more drugs. Because some people's medical conditions will improve over the passage of time or by chance, the researchers must show that the improvement seen is caused by the treatment. Some benefits or risks of a drug may not appear for several years, so participants are often contacted by the researchers long after the study has ended.

The size of studies designed to identify the best treatments is especially critical. If too few people are tested, researchers will not know whether the results of the study will apply to the general population. Neither will they know whether a treatment proved better only by chance.

QUESTIONS ASKED IN HYPERTENSION STUDIES

For antihypertensive (blood pressure–lowering) drugs and lifestyle changes, researchers ask two basic questions: Does the treatment lower blood pressure? Does the treatment prevent strokes and heart attacks?

The first question is straightforward. Researchers compare blood pressure readings taken before and after treatment in all groups. Comparing these numbers gives a clear answer to the question of effectiveness. This question is easily answered and is rarely the focus of a clinical trial.

Whether a hypertension treatment prevents stroke and heart attack is actually the more important question. Lowering blood pressure is known to reduce stroke risk, but it does not necessarily reduce heart attack risk. This second question has been answered for only weight loss and use of beta blockers: these treatments have been proven to reduce both blood pressure and the risk of stroke and heart attack. Research has also shown that diuretics help prevent heart attacks in most people. While newer drugs and other lifestyle changes (such as regular exercise) are known to lower blood pressure, their long-term effects in preventing heart attack have not yet been proved. Some medications offer additional protection against heart disease by lowering low density lipoprotein (LDL, or "bad") cholesterol levels. Others have negative effects that may offset their benefits.

Other concerns addressed by hypertension studies relate to other health risks and quality of life. Does the treatment increase cholesterol levels or insulin resistance? Does it lower them? Does the drug interfere with a person's usual daily routine? Does the treatment cause more problems than it solves? (This is particularly important when assessing the side effects of single drugs or drug combinations.)

For example, the Systolic Hypertension in the Elderly Program (SHEP) was conducted to determine if antihypertensive drugs reduced the number of fatal and nonfatal cardiovascular events (such as heart attacks) in older adults with hypertension. The study also assessed the effects of the medication on thinking ability, mood, or routine activities. The 4,736 patients received either a diuretic–beta blocker combination (chlorthalidone/atenolol) or a placebo and were monitored for 5 years. SHEP conclusively showed that active treatment significantly lowered the number of strokes and deaths. Side effects, including memory impairment, were reported by an almost equal proportion of participants in both groups. Participants in the placebo group actually had more difficulty completing their usual activities of daily living than those taking the active drugs.

SHOULD YOU JOIN A CLINICAL TRIAL?

If you live near a research hospital or university, you may have read or heard advertisements for clinical trials. Today, most clinical trials examining hypertension treatment are past the early experimental stage and now seek to determine which treatment is best at preventing heart attacks and strokes. Drug companies studying new medications not yet approved by the US Food and Drug Administration (USFDA) make this clear, so that you can make an informed decision whether to participate.

Participants often receive much more thorough health care than they usually receive. This extra care comes at no expense to the participant. The medications are always free, as are any medical tests and doctor visits related specifically to the study. In most trials, if your blood pressure goes up, the doctor will adjust your treatment to control your hypertension. Your medical information is shared with your personal physician. All of the benefits and risks of joining a study are explained to you when you first go in. Perhaps the best reason for joining a clinical trial is the benefit you will provide to other people, possibly your own children.

If you hear of a study that you would like to join, ask your doctor about it, and then contact the organization that is conducting the study for more information. Usually, studies have eligibility requirements. That is, they may not be able to take you if you have another disease, are too old or too young, have blood pressure that is too high or too low, are planning to become pregnant during the course of the study, are taking a certain drug, or are unusual or unique in some other way. Remember, many of these studies seek to find the best treatments for the broadest possible population. Researchers also do not want to put you at risk for additional disease. Often, the researchers can determine whether you are eligible for the study by asking questions, but you may also need to give a blood sample or urine sample.

Most studies require that you be able to travel to the research clinic, but a few will allow you to see your personal physician, who sends in your information. Some organizations try to make study participation more convenient by paying for parking or transportation, but you cannot always count on this, especially in very large studies. Usually, they will try to accommodate your work schedule and daily routine. You will probably have forms to fill out at home, and you will need to return to the research clinic at regular intervals. Studies that involve some sort of lifestyle change often provide support groups and educational meetings to help you modify your diet, increase your activity level, or lose weight.

CURRENT HYPERTENSION STUDIES

Many hypertension studies are being conducted around the world. Some focus on specific populations, such as African Americans or older adults. Others restrict themselves to a certain drug or class of drugs, such as calcium channel blockers. The researchers who plan and run clinical trials often assign them names that can be more easily remembered by their acronyms, such as the Antihypertensive and Lipid-Lowering Treatment to Prevent Heart Attack Trial (ALLHAT) or the African American Study of Kidney Disease and Hypertension (AASK). Here is a description of some current hypertension studies.

ALLHAT. ALLHAT is sponsored by the National Heart, Lung, and Blood Institute (NHLBI), which is part of the National Institutes of Health (NIH), in conjunction with the Department of Veterans Affairs. ALLHAT is the largest clinical trial studying hypertension ever conducted in the US. It will also study more African Americans and people with diabetes than any previous hypertension trial. Eligible patients are 55 years and older with diagnosed hypertension who also have at least one additional risk factor for cardiovascular disease (such as smoking, left ventricular hypertrophy, low levels of high density lipoprotein [HDL, or "good"] cholesterol, or high levels of low density lipoprotein [LDL, or "bad"] cholesterol). ALLHAT enrolled participants through its research centers, community hospitals, health maintenance organizations (HMOs), and most notably, private practices (which account for about 40 percent of the research sites).

This randomized, double-blind study has been designed to answer two questions. First, ALLHAT will determine whether newer types of antihypertensive drugs, which may be more costly to purchase, are as good as or better than diuretics in reducing the incidence or severity of coronary artery disease. For this, the study will measure the effectiveness of four drugs in the prevention of strokes and heart attacks: a diuretic (chlorthalidone), a calcium channel blocker (amlodipine), an ACE inhibitor (lisinopril), and an alpha blocker (doxazosin). The trial has enrolled 40,000 patients over the age of 55 who will be monitored for at least 5 years. Second, ALLHAT will determine if lowering LDL cholesterol in older people with elevated cholesterol levels can reduce cardiovascular disease and death. Half of the patients in the main study will be enrolled in a randomized trial and given either pravastatin (a cholesterol-lowering drug) or a placebo in addition to their blood pressure medication. People were enrolled in the study between 1994 and January 1998 and will be monitored for 5 to 7 years.

AASK. This study is being funded by the NIH. African Americans are susceptible to kidney damage from hypertension (see Chapter 3), and this study is designed to answer two questions:

What is the optimal level of blood pressure for preventing kidney damage? Which of three types of medication (a beta blocker, a calcium channel blocker, or an ACE inhibitor) is best? Kidney function will be assessed throughout the study, which will last from 4 to 7 years. AASK began in 1995 and is expected to be completed by 2002.

Hypertension Optimal Treatment Study. An ongoing study that is nearing completion, the Hypertension Optimal Treatment (HOT) study includes 19,000 patients in the US and 25 other countries. The study is sponsored by the drug companies Astra USA and Astra Merck. The study's goal is to determine how low the blood pressure should be kept to minimize the occurrence of strokes and heart attacks. Participants are randomized into three treatment groups, each with different target diastolic blood pressure levels: below 80 mm Hg, below 85 mm Hg, and below 90 mm Hg. Enrollment is complete, and the participants are being monitored for 3 years. At this writing, it appears that the results of the study may be known in 1998.

WHEN YOU HEAR ABOUT MEDICAL STUDIES IN THE NEWS . . .

More and more, you hear about the latest medical advances on the evening news or read about them in the headlines in the morning paper. The studies mentioned above will probably receive a mention of some sort in the popular press. And so will smaller, less rigorous studies. How do you know which headlines to believe? What do you do when one study says one thing but another study says something else? How do you decide when the results of one study will affect your own treatment?

None of these questions is easy to answer. Too often, important details that may help you determine the value of a study's results are left out of news reports. Before you panic or rejoice at the latest medical news, be sure to gather as many facts as you can so that you can talk to your doctor and ask informed questions.

Usually, even the briefest news report will indicate who is sponsoring the study. Government health agencies or large public health organizations generally produce the most widely respected study results. Many drug companies also conduct large, well-controlled trials. You can consider the study sponsor in light of other details (such as study size, type, and duration) when deciding whether the study was truly scientific.

You can use the information about clinical trials outlined above to determine whether a given study is likely to offer accurate, unbiased information about treatment. Consider whether the study was randomized, controlled, or blind. Look at the number of participants in each treatment group; a study of only 8, 9, 20, or 40 people probably is not conclusive—even if the topic grabs headline attention. Notice how long participants were monitored and what outcomes were measured (such as blood pressure, cholesterol levels, number of strokes, number of heart attacks, and number of deaths).

Finally, ask yourself if the results of the study matter in real life. If one drug is better than another, how much better is it? You may not benefit from a 1- to 2-mm Hg improvement in your blood pressure. Also, certain lifestyle changes, such as a strict vegetarian diet, are too drastic to be useful to many people. You might be better off making more moderate changes to your diet that you can stick with for the rest of your life—for example, increasing the number of servings of fruits and vegetables you eat each day. Were the participants like you? A study limited to one age group, one ethnic group, or one sex is irrelevant if your profile does not match that of the typical participant.

It is usually unwise and sometimes dangerous to allow the results of one study to convince you to change your medication or lifestyle. Look for advice from government organizations (such as the NHLBI), major public health organizations (such as the AMA and the American Heart Association [AHA]), and your physician.

16

Common Questions and Answers About Hypertension

Q. **If I have hypertension, why do I feel good?**

A. Some people think their blood pressure is high only when they are flushed, angry, tense, or excited. And their blood pressure may in fact be slightly elevated at those times. However, in most cases, hypertension produces no obvious symptoms. Because of this, it is often called "the silent killer" (see Chapter 3).

Q. **Will I have high blood pressure for the rest of my life?**

A. If your high blood pressure is caused by an underlying disease (secondary hypertension), your blood pressure should return to normal after the underlying disease is successfully treated. However, this is not true for essential (or primary) hypertension (high blood pressure with no known cause). Since there is no cure for essential hypertension, you will always have it, even when your blood pressure has been brought under control with lifestyle changes and medication. But by working closely with your doctor to keep your blood pressure under control, you can significantly reduce your risk of stroke, heart attack, heart failure, and kidney failure, and improve your chances of living a normal, healthy life.

Q. **How can my kidneys be causing hypertension? I thought hypertension was a heart disease.**

A. In some people, hypertension occurs when the artery that brings blood to the kidney (the renal artery) becomes narrowed or blocked. This type of hypertension is called renovascular hypertension (see Chapter 2). In an attempt to increase blood flow, the kidney releases an enzyme called renin, which starts a chemical chain reaction that results in higher blood pressure. Renovascular hypertension can sometimes be treated by opening up the affected renal artery through surgery or angioplasty.

Q. **I just checked the blood pressure in my other arm and got a different reading. Should I see my doctor?**

A. Most people have a slightly different blood pressure in each arm. Small differences in readings taken from both arms at the same sitting are normal. However, if your blood pressure is consistently 10 mm Hg or more higher in one arm than in the other, you should see your doctor. The difference in blood pressure could be a sign of atherosclerosis (narrowing of an artery caused by buildup of fatty deposits on the artery wall).

Q. **I heard that salt intake does not matter anymore. Is this true?**

A. The amount of salt in the diet is a problem only for those people with hypertension who are salt sensitive. When people who are salt sensitive eat too much salt (sodium), their blood pressure goes up. This is particularly common among African Americans and older people of all racial and ethnic backgrounds. Ask your doctor if you should cut back on salt.

Q. **I have high blood pressure. Is it safe for me to exercise?**

A. For most people, regular exercise actually helps lower blood pressure (see Chapter 6). Research has shown that exercising at a moderate level (that is, so that you can talk comfortably while exercising) for at least 30 minutes three or four times per week can lower blood pressure by about 5 to 10 mm Hg. However, it is a good idea to avoid exercising within 2 to 3 hours of eating a meal, particularly if you regularly experience angina. If it is controlled, your high blood pressure does not put you at any special risk during moderate exercise, but another condition, such as left ventricular hypertrophy, could possibly cause problems. In any case, be sure to talk with your doctor before starting an exercise program or significantly increasing your usual level of activity.

Q. **Should I switch to decaffeinated coffee?**

A. Research shows that caffeine temporarily raises blood pressure and heart rate by a small amount in most people. If you feel palpitations (an abnormally strong, rapid heartbeat) or skipped heartbeats, you may want to switch to decaffeinated coffee to eliminate these unpleasant symptoms. If your hypertension is especially severe, your doctor may recommend that you avoid all caffeinated beverages, including tea and some soft drinks, such as colas. Also, it is a good idea to avoid drinking or eating anything that contains caffeine shortly before having a blood pressure check, since this may cause an inaccurate reading. Ask your doctor if you need to avoid caffeine.

Q. **My blood pressure went down when I took medication, and I thought that was the end of the problem. Do these drugs cure hypertension?**

A. No. Hypertension cannot be cured in most people. As discussed in Chapter 2, only in people in whom a treatable medical condition causes hypertension can blood pressure be lowered permanently (by treating the underlying cause). If lifestyle changes do not lower your blood pressure sufficiently, then medication is needed to help prevent health problems caused by uncontrolled high blood pressure (see Chapter 3). Antihypertensive medications work only for a certain length of time, usually no more than 24 hours, and must therefore be taken every day. Normal or lowered blood pressure readings indicate that your medication is working the way it is supposed to work. If you stop taking your medication exactly as your doctor prescribed, your blood pressure will go back up.

Q. **I feel fine except when I take my medication. Can I skip a dose occasionally?**

A. No. As explained above, antihypertensive medications must be taken exactly as prescribed to help control blood pressure. Otherwise, you will be at risk for many health problems (see Chapter 3), including atherosclerosis (narrowing of the arteries caused by buildup of fatty deposits on artery walls), kidney disease, vision problems, heart attack, or stroke. If your medication is causing unpleasant side effects, talk with your doctor. He or she can adjust or change your medication so that your blood pressure is controlled without unpleasant side effects.

Q. **A coworker of mine is very happy with the antihypertensive drug she is taking. Should I switch medications?**

A. No. Her doctor chose her medication after considering many factors specific to her alone. Your doctor considered your health history, age, race, other medical conditions, laboratory test results, and other important factors when selecting the medication you take. If you are unhappy with your current medication for any reason, talk to your doctor and explain your concerns. And never take medication prescribed for another person.

Q. **Why do some drugs have so many different names?**

A. New drugs are always listed by a brand name, given by the manufacturer, and a generic (chemical) name. When the patent secured by the drug company that developed a particular medication runs out (17 years after the patent was awarded), any drug manufacturer can then produce the drug. Therefore, antihypertensive drugs that have been used for more than 17 years may have several brand names for the same generic drug. For example, the diuretic hydrochlorothiazide (generic name) is sold as Esidrix by Novartis, as HydroDIURIL by Merck, and as Oretic by Abbott.

Q. **My doctor said that I may have a problem with postural hypotension because of my medication. What is that?**

A. Hypotension is the opposite of hypertension and refers to very low blood pressure. Postural hypotension occurs when you move quickly from a sitting or lying position. Your blood pressure drops suddenly, and you feel faint or dizzy. You may actually lose consciousness. This occurs because your blood pressure is too low to get enough blood to your brain. If this happens to you, be sure to tell your doctor as soon as possible. To treat this condition, your doctor may change or adjust your blood pressure medication, perhaps by lowering the dose or altering the combination of drugs you are taking. You can help prevent symptoms yourself by remembering always to get up slowly from a lying or sitting position. In older adults and people with diabetes, postural hypotension can also indicate a more serious problem in the body's mechanisms for regulating blood pressure and may need to be examined more closely.

Q. I think my blood pressure goes up only at the doctor's office. Could this be my problem?

A. Perhaps, at least in part. About one of every five people with hypertension has a problem called "white coat hypertension." In these people, blood pressure rises when they are in a doctor's office, clinic, or other health facility. Sometimes waiting and relaxing a while before having your blood pressure checked will help reduce the likelihood of getting an artificially elevated reading. Some clinics have found that having a health-care professional in street clothes checking blood pressures helps eliminate the problem. If you feel that your blood pressure is high only at your doctor's office, you can confirm this yourself by checking your blood pressure at home. In some cases, your doctor may recommend that you wear a special blood pressure monitor for several days that will record how much your blood pressure fluctuates throughout the day and show whether it is at a healthy level most of the time.

Q. Medication is so expensive, and I do not have health insurance, or my insurance covers only part of the cost. What can I do?

A. First, make sure you have made lifestyle changes that could lower your blood pressure without the need for drugs. Weight loss, regular exercise, a balanced diet low in fat and sodium, and stress management are just a few of the self-help treatments that can lower high blood pressure. (Chapter 6 reviews these in detail.)

Second, if you need to take medication to control your blood pressure, remember that the cost of the drugs will, over the long run, be much less than the cost of your medical treatment if you have a heart attack, stroke, kidney failure, or other serious health problem caused by your hypertension. Ask your doctor whether one of the less expensive types of drugs (diuretics or beta blockers, discussed in Chapter 8) would work for you.

Third, the price of medicines varies greatly among pharmacies. If cost is a problem, ask your doctor or pharmacist if there is a lower-cost generic form of your medicine available. Sometimes the same drug manufacturer produces both a brand-name and a generic form of the same medication. You can also compare prices at different pharmacies and mail-order prescription services.

Finally, if it is needed, financial assistance may be available through social service agencies in your community. You also may qualify for help through prescription assistance programs established by certain drug companies. Let your doctor know if the cost of medication is a problem. He or she may be able to help you apply for assistance or advise you where to apply. The Resources section of this book shows you how to get information about some of these programs.

Q. **I just found out that I am pregnant, and I do not want to hurt the baby. Should I stop taking my medication until I see my doctor?**

A. No. Controlling your blood pressure is more important to your baby's health than the possible effects of your antihypertensive medication. Most blood pressure drugs are safe to use during pregnancy (see Chapter 12). Your doctor probably prescribed one of these, especially if you indicated that you might become pregnant. If you are taking an angiotensin converting enzyme (ACE) inhibitor, you will need to change drugs early in your pregnancy and should talk to your doctor about switching medications—but do not stop taking your medication until your doctor tells you to stop. While antihypertensive medications are safe and necessary during pregnancy and will not prevent you from breastfeeding your baby, dosages may need to be adjusted as your pregnancy continues and again after delivery.

Q. **Both my husband and I have hypertension. How often should we have our children checked?**

A. Some children may inherit a tendency toward high blood pressure from their parents. This is especially true in African American families. If you and your husband have hypertension, your doctor should check each child's blood pressure once a year. As a family, you should all be engaging in heart-healthy habits, such as a low-fat, low-sodium diet, regular physical activity, and no smoking or alcohol consumption. Since your children are at risk for developing hypertension even earlier than you or your husband did, these lifestyle changes are particularly important for preventing high blood pressure and other cardiovascular disease.

Q. What is the best way to get ready for a visit to my doctor?

A. The best way to get ready for a visit to your doctor is to write down any questions you want to ask and prepare a list of any unusual symptoms you may have (including drug side effects). Bring a record of blood pressure readings if you are monitoring your own blood pressure at home. Also, bring a list of all the medications you are currently taking, including vitamins and nonprescription drugs. Preparing for your visit in advance will help you stay focused and ensure that all of your questions and concerns are addressed.

Q. I sometimes forget to take my blood pressure medication. What can I do to remember?

A. A good way to remember to take your medication is to make it part of your daily routine. Taking your medication at the same time every day, such as just before a meal or after you brush your teeth, will help you remember to take it. You may also find it useful to mark your calendar with a check or some other notation so that you can easily keep track. The routine of marking your calendar should also help you to remember. If you take your blood pressure medication with other drugs, you may want to purchase a medication organizer, a box with spaces for days of the week. Some even have alarms to remind you to take your medication at specific times; or you could set an alarm to go off daily on a digital watch or a clock as a reminder. You can also enlist the help of family or other household members to remind you when it is time to take your medications.

Resources

The organizations listed below can provide you with the latest information about high blood pressure and associated health problems. Some groups offer free information, and some offer books or other materials for sale to consumers. Most have toll-free numbers to call and information sites on the worldwide web. All telephone numbers refer to voice communication except those designed (as noted) for use by people who are hearing impaired (telecommunication device for the deaf, or TDD) or by facsimile machines (fax).

American Academy of Family Physicians (AAFP)
8880 Ward Parkway
Kansas City, MO 64114
phone: (800) 274-2237 or (816) 333-9700

WEB SITE:
http://www.aafp.org

> The AAFP is a nonprofit medical association of family physicians—the type of doctor most likely to treat people with hypertension. The academy offers patient information handouts, brochures, and a newsletter.

American Academy of Pediatrics (AAP)
141 Northwest Point Boulevard
P.O. Box 927
Elk Grove Village, IL 60007-0927
phone: (847) 228-5005
fax: (847) 228-5097

WEB SITE:
http://www.aap.org

The AAP is a professional organization dedicated to the health, safety, and well-being of infants, children, and young adults. The academy publishes books, brochures, and much more on child and adolescent health topics both for health-care professionals and for the general public.

American College of Cardiology (ACC)
9111 Old Georgetown Road
Bethesda, MD 20814-1699
phone: (800) 253-4636 or (301) 897-5400
fax: (301) 897-9745

WEB SITE:
  http://www.acc.org

Your personal physician will treat your hypertension. However, you may need to see a heart specialist, a cardiologist, if you have complications related to your high blood pressure or other heart disease. The ACC is a professional society of cardiovascular doctors and scientists from all over the world. To become a member, doctors must have special knowledge and experience in treating heart disorders. The college offers patient education materials and referrals to board certified cardiologists.

American Diabetes Association (ADA)
1660 Duke Street
Alexandria, VA 22314
phone: (800) 232-3472 or (703) 549-1500

WEB SITE:
  http://www.diabetes.org

The ADA was created to fight diabetes through education and research. Local affiliates offer patient education services, and the ADA publishes materials on a wide variety of topics of interest to people with diabetes.

American Dietetic Association (ADA)
216 West Jackson Boulevard, 7th floor
Chicago, IL 60606-6995
phone: (800) 366-1655 or (312) 899-0040

WEB SITE:

http://www.eatright.org

The ADA promotes the science of nutrition and public education about foods, nutrition, and health. You can call the ADA nutrition hotline for recorded messages about diet and health or to speak with a registered dietitian. The ADA also publishes nutrition information in a wide variety of formats.

American Heart Association (AHA)
National Center
7272 Greenville Avenue
Dallas, TX 75231-4596
phone: (800) 242-8721 or (214) 373-6300

WEB SITE:

http://www.amhrt.org

The AHA, a nonprofit, voluntary health agency, is dedicated to the reduction of death and disability from cardiovascular disease, including heart disease and stroke. Local chapters offer public education programs, and the AHA publishes information on all aspects of hypertension and other cardiovascular disease, including brochures targeted at special groups (such as African Americans, older adults, and children).

American Medical Association (AMA)
515 North State Street
Chicago, IL 60610
phone: (312) 464-5000

WEB SITE:

http://www.ama-assn.org

The American Medical Association serves doctors and their patients by promoting ethical, educational, and clinical standards for the medical profession. Research on hypertension, atherosclerosis, and related topics is often published in the *Journal of the American Medical Association* (*JAMA*) or other scientific journals. The AMA publishes health information and medical news for consumers and physicians; also it provides referrals to licensed doctors in the US via county medical societies.

Canadian Hypertension Society (CHS)
c/o Department of Pharmacology
Room A329, Chown Building
University of Manitoba
753 McDermot Avenue
Winnipeg, Manitoba R3E 0T6
phone: (204) 789-3356

WEB SITE:
http://www.umanitoba.ca/outreach/chs

The Canadian Hypertension Society is a nonprofit organization affiliated with the Royal College of Physicians and Surgeons of Canada. The CHS produces a quarterly newsletter to promote awareness of hypertension research and offers free educational literature to the public.

Canadian Medical Association
1867 Alta Vista Drive
Ottawa, ON
K1G 3Y6
phone: (613) 731-9331

WEB SITE:
http://www.cma.ca

The Canadian Medical Association is a valuable source of medical information and resources. The group's web site contains a search engine that will help you locate links to specific medical topics, including hypertension.

CenterWatch, Inc.
581 Boylston Street
Boston, MA 02116
phone: (617) 247-2327
fax: (617) 247-2535

WEB SITE:

http://www.centerwatch.com

CenterWatch is a clinical trials listing service from which you can get information about clinical trials and newly approved drugs, including generic equivalents, that have come on the market. On the worldwide web, you can search for a particular clinical trial, be notified via e-mail about new trials recruiting participants, and read about the medical centers conducting research.

Citizens for Public Action on High Blood Pressure and Cholesterol
P.O. Box 30374
Bethesda, MD 20824
phone: (301) 770-1711

Citizens for Public Action on High Blood Pressure and Cholesterol is a nonprofit advocacy group for public policy and resources to prevent heart disease. The group publishes a series of brochures related to blood pressure and cholesterol, as well as a newsletter.

Health Canada
A.L. 0913A
Ottawa, Canada
K1A OK9
phone: (613) 941-5336

WEB SITE:

http://www.hc-sc.gc.ca

Health Canada is the federal department responsible for helping Canadians maintain their health. The department promotes disease prevention and healthy living. You can search Health Canada's medical database for information on specific health-related topics.

HeartInfo
Center for Cardiovascular Education, Inc.
P.O. Box 823
New Providence, NJ 07974-0823
phone: (908) 665-4153

WEB SITE:
   http://www.heartinfo.org

   HeartInfo is an independent, educational worldwide web site dedicated to providing information and services to people with any sort of cardiovascular disorder. The site is geared toward consumers and is managed by Daniel James Rader, MD, Director of the Lipid Referral Center and the Cardiovascular Risk Intervention Program at the University of Pennsylvania Health System. You will find material about heart disease, the latest news on treatment options, and information on available products and services.

Heart Information Service
Texas Heart Institute
P.O. Box 20345
Houston, TX 77225-0345
phone: (800) 292-2221 or (713) 794-6630
fax: (713) 794-3714

   The Heart Information Service, a program of the Texas Heart Institute, is a national hotline that answers questions from the general public regarding the diagnosis, treatment, and prevention of cardiovascular disease.

The Heart: An Online Exploration

WEB SITE:
   http://www.fi.edu/biosci.heart.html

   The Franklin Institute in Philadelphia, Pennsylvania, offers an online, multimedia tour of your cardiovascular system. You will be able to see how your heart and blood vessels work, learn more about your kidneys and lungs, monitor your own heart's health, and look back on the history of heart science. This worldwide web site is especially good for people looking for a basic understanding of their heart and circulatory system and for parents teaching their children about their heart and heart disease risks.

Hypertension Network, Inc.
P.O. Box 302
Wingdale, NY 12594

WEB SITE:

http://www.bloodpressure.com

The Hypertension Network, Inc., headed by Thomas Pickering, MD, DPhil, aims to improve the quality of medical care available to people with high blood pressure. The network answers questions about the disorder and its treatment, provides updated information on available drugs, and reviews products available for people with hypertension.

National Clearinghouse for Alcohol and Drug Information
P.O. Box 2345
Rockville, MD 20847-2345
phone: (800) 729-6686 or (800) 487-4889 (telecommunication device for the deaf [TDD])
fax: (301) 468-6433

WEB SITE:

http://www.health.org

Prevention Online (PREVLINE) is a service of the National Clearinghouse for Alcohol and Drug Information. The clearinghouse is the largest resource for current information and materials about substance abuse (including alcohol and tobacco).

National Council on the Aging, Inc.
409 3rd Street, SW
Washington, D.C. 20024
phone: (202) 479-1200
fax: (202) 479-0735

WEB SITE:

http://www.ncoa.org

The National Council on the Aging, Inc. is a private, nonprofit organization that serves as a resource for information, technical assistance, advocacy, and leadership in all aspects of aging. A large number of brochures are available on topics of interest to older Americans, their families, and health-care professionals.

National Health Information Center
P.O. Box 1133
Washington, D.C. 20013-1133
phone: (800) 336-4797 or (301) 565-4167
fax: (301) 984-4256

WEB SITE:
  http://nhic–nt.health.org

> The National Health Information Center helps people locate health
> information through an enormous database of health organizations
> and the resources they offer. If you are not sure which health or
> medical organization to contact for specific information, check here
> first.

National Heart, Lung, and Blood Institute Information Center
P.O. Box 30105
Bethesda, MD 20824-0105
phone: (301) 251-1222
recorded heart health information: (800) 575-9355
fax: (301) 251-1223

WEB SITE:
  http://www.nhlbi.nih.gov

> The National Heart, Lung, and Blood Institute Information Center
> seeks to improve public health by translating the results of medical
> research into practical consumer advice. The information center
> serves as a clearinghouse for brochures, posters, audiovisual mate-
> rials, cookbooks, and many more materials important to people
> with hypertension and heart disease.

National Institute of Diabetes and Digestive and Kidney Disease
1 Information Way
Bethesda, MD 20892-3560

WEB SITE:
  http://www.niddk.nih.gov

> The National Institute of Diabetes and Digestive and Kidney Dis-
> ease offers information to the general public on a wide variety of

topics of interest to people with hypertension: diabetes, kidney disease, weight control, and nutrition.

National Institute of Neurologic Disorders and Stroke
Office of Scientific and Health Reports
31 Center Drive, MSC 2540, building 31, room 8A-06
Bethesda, MD 20892-2540
phone: (301) 496-5751
fax: (301) 402-2186

WEB SITE:
http://www.ninds.nih.gov

The National Institute of Neurologic Disorders and Stroke conducts and supports research on the causes, prevention, diagnosis, and treatment of stroke and other disorders of the brain and nervous system. Consumer publications on a variety of topics are available.

National Institute on Aging Information Center
P.O. Box 8057
Gaithersburg, MD 20898-8057
phone: (800) 222-2225 or (800) 222-4225 (TDD)

WEB SITES:
http://www.nih.gov/nia/
http://www.aoa.dhhs.gov/

The National Institute on Aging publishes more than 60 free brochures and a series of fact sheets called Age Pages covering a large number of health topics of interest to older adults.

National Kidney Foundation
30 East 33rd Street
New York, NY 10016
phone: (800) 622-9010 or (212) 889-2210

WEB SITE:
http://www.kidney.org

The National Kidney Foundation, directly and through its affiliates, publishes pamphlets on kidney disease and offers health screening, counseling, referrals, transportation, and other programs for people with kidney disease.

National Stroke Association
96 Inverness Drive East, suite 1
Englewood, CO 80112-5112
phone: (800) 787-6537 or (303) 649-9299
fax: (303) 649-1328

WEB SITE:
  http://www.stroke.org

The National Stroke Association is a nonprofit organization dedicated to educating stroke survivors, families, health-care professionals, and the general public about stroke. The association offers information and referrals and provides guidance on establishing stroke support groups.

Office of Minority Health Resource Center
P.O. Box 37337
Washington, D.C. 20013-7337
phone: (800) 444-6472 or (301) 589-0951
fax: (301) 589-0884

WEB SITE:
  http://www.omhrc.gov

The Office of Minority Health Resource Center responds to questions and requests for information related to minority health concerns and provides referrals to appropriate organizations. Staff members can serve people who speak Spanish.

Office on Smoking and Health
National Center for Chronic Disease Prevention and Health Promotion
Centers for Disease Control and Prevention (CDC)
Mail Stop K-50
4770 Buford Highway, NE

Atlanta, GA 30341-3724
phone: (800) 232-1311 or (770) 488-5705
fax: (770) 488-5939

WEB SITE:
  http://www.cdc.gov/nccdphp/osh/tobacco.html

> The National Center for Chronic Disease Prevention and Health Promotion offers a wide variety of materials and information useful for people with hypertension. The Office on Smoking and Health provides publications on smoking and health as well as smoking cessation support.

NEWSGROUP:
  sci.med.cardiology

> This Usenet newsgroup on the internet discusses topics related to cardiovascular disease. While much of the discussion is technical in nature and serves basically as an opportunity for cardiologists (doctors who specialize in heart disease) to exchange their thoughts and experiences, you may find some useful information here. However, as with all medical information obtained over the internet, do not follow any health advice until you discuss it with your doctor. Some of the information and advice may be inaccurate or misleading, or it may not apply to your situation because of factors in your personal health history. You may also want to post questions related to your blood pressure management at **sci.med.nursing** (another Usenet newsgroup used mainly by nurses but open to questions from the general public) and questions related to your medications at **sci.med.pharmacy** (used by pharmacists).

Women's Health America Group
P.O. Box 259690
Madison, WI 53725
phone: (800) 558-7046
fax: (888) 898-7412

> The Women's Health America Group is a national organization designed to serve the unique and complex health needs of women by providing current, accurate health information.

Women's Health Initiative
7550 Rockville Pike, Federal Building, room 6A-09
Bethesda, MD 20892-9110
phone: (301) 402-2900

WEB SITE:

http://whi.nih.gov

The Women's Health Initiative is a 15-year research program designed to study the major causes of death and disability in women and to reduce coronary heart disease, breast and colon cancer, and osteoporosis in postmenopausal women.

Glossary

This glossary defines terms that your doctor may have mentioned or that you may have come across while reading about hypertension. Italicized words within entries refer you to other entries in this section for additional information.

A

abdominal angina: Abdominal pain that occurs when the blood supply to the intestines is insufficient, usually due to blockage of the arteries. Abdominal angina is worse after meals and often occurs at a fixed time after eating.

accelerated hypertension: A condition in which significantly elevated *blood pressure* is accompanied by damage to the blood vessels in the back of the eye. Accelerated hypertension can quickly progress to *malignant hypertension* if not treated.

ACE (angiotensin converting enzyme) inhibitor: A type of medication that lowers *blood pressure* by blocking the action of *angiotensin converting enzyme (ACE)*.

acromegaly: A condition marked by progressive enlargement of the hands, face, feet, and chest caused by a disorder in the pituitary gland. In very rare cases, this can be the cause of *hypertension*.

adrenal gland: A chemical-producing organ that releases several *hormones*, including *aldosterone*, cortisol, *epinephrine*, and *norepinephrine*. There are two adrenal glands, one on top of each *kidney*. Tumors in the adrenal glands can cause *hypertension*.

adrenaline: See *epinephrine*.

adrenergic: Related to nerve cells that release the hormone *norepinephrine* as a *neurotransmitter*.

albuminuria: The presence of too much protein in the urine, which usually indicates disease.

aldosterone: A *hormone* released by the *adrenal glands* that causes the *kidneys* to retain *sodium* and to eliminate *potassium,* raising *blood pressure.*

aldosteronism: A condition in which too much *aldosterone* is released by the *adrenal glands.* One symptom of this condition is *hypertension.*

alpha blocker: A type of medication that dilates (widens) the arteries by blocking *norepinephrine* from reaching the *alpha receptors* on arterial walls.

alpha receptor: A protein on the wall of an *artery* into which *norepinephrine* fits like a key into a lock. When triggered by norepinephrine, alpha receptors cause the blood vessels to contract, raising *blood pressure.*

aneurysm: Balloonlike expansion of a blood vessel caused by a weakening of the vessel wall. An aneurysm can burst, causing a *stroke* (in the brain) or hemorrhage elsewhere in the body.

angina pectoris: Chest pain that occurs when the heart does not receive enough blood. This type of pain is often a symptom of *coronary artery* disease. Early in the disease, angina pectoris may occur only during exertion or strong emotions, but later it can occur even while the person is at rest. Angina pectoris is often called simply angina.

angiography: A procedure for examining blood vessels in which dye is injected and X rays are taken to show whether blood passes through or is blocked by plaque.

angioplasty: A procedure in which a laser, a balloon catheter, or surgery is used to open blocked *coronary arteries.*

angiotensin: An inactive protein circulating in the blood that can be split by *angiotensin converting enzyme (ACE)* to form *angiotensin II.*

angiotensin II: An active *hormone* formed when *angiotensin converting enzyme (ACE)* acts on *angiotensin* to split it in two. Angiotensin II causes blood vessels to contract, raising *blood pressure,* and stimulates the *adrenal glands* to release *aldosterone,* which also contributes to *hypertension.*

angiotensin blockers: A type of medication that blocks the action of *angiotensin II* on blood vessels and the *adrenal glands.*

angiotensin converting enzyme (ACE): A protein required to convert *angiotensin* to *angiotensin II,* which can cause the arteries to constrict, raising *blood pressure.*

antioxidant: A substance that helps protect the body from damage caused by *free radicals.* Antioxidants are produced in the body and are found in many foods, especially fruits and vegetables; antioxidant supplements are also available.

aorta: The body's main artery, which carries blood away from the heart to the rest of the body.

arrhythmia: A condition in which the normal, regular rhythm of the heartbeat is disturbed.

arteriole: A small branch of an artery that connects to a *capillary.*

arteriosclerosis: Hardening of the arteries that occurs naturally with age or as a result of *atherosclerosis.*

artery: A blood vessel that carries oxygenated blood away from the heart to the tissues of the body. The one exception is the pulmonary artery, which carries deoxygenated blood from the heart to the lungs.

atherectomy: A surgical procedure for opening blocked *coronary arteries* with a tiny rotating shaver that removes the plaque lining the arterial walls.

atherosclerosis: A type of *arteriosclerosis* in which deposits (called plaques) of fatty substances, cellular waste products, calcium, and clotting material build up on the inner lining of an artery, thereby narrowing the passage and reducing blood flow.

autonomic nervous system: The branch of the central nervous system that regulates involuntary body functions, such as respiration, digestion, and the circulation of blood. The autonomic nervous system is divided into the *sympathetic nervous system* and the parasympathetic nervous system.

B

beta blocker: A type of medication that reduces the force and rate of the heartbeat to lower *blood pressure* and to treat *angina pectoris* resulting from *coronary artery* disease. Beta blockers work by preventing *norepinephrine* from acting on *beta receptors* on the heart and *kidneys.*

beta receptor: A protein on the wall of the heart and *kidneys* into which *norepinephrine* fits like a key into a lock. When triggered by norepinephrine, beta receptors cause the heart to beat faster and the kidneys to produce *renin*, both of which raise *blood pressure*.

blood pressure: The force of blood against the walls of the arteries. Blood pressure is created by two opposing forces, that of the heart beating and that of the arteries resisting blood flow.

blood volume: The total amount of blood circulating in the *cardiovascular* system.

bruit: An abnormal sound heard when a *stethoscope* is placed over an *artery*, often indicating a blockage.

C

calcium channel blocker: A type of medication that interferes with the movement of calcium in and out of the blood vessel wall. When calcium cannot flow into the cells, the blood vessels dilate (widen).

capillary: The smallest type of blood vessel in the body, only a single cell wide, responsible for delivering oxygen and nutrients to individual cells. The capillaries link *arterioles*, from which they receive oxygenated blood, and venules, to which they send waste products collected from the cells.

cardiac output: The amount of blood pumped by the heart in 1 minute.

cardiovascular: Refers to the heart and blood vessels (*arteries*, *veins*, and *capillaries*).

carotid arteries: The large *arteries* in the neck that supply blood to the brain.

CAT scan: See *computed tomography* (*CT*) *scanning*.

catecholamine: A type of *hormone* released by the *sympathetic nervous system*. *Epinephrine* and *norepinephrine* are catecholamines.

cerebral: Refers to the brain.

cholesterol: A soft, waxy substance found among the *lipids* in the blood and in every cell in the body. Cholesterol is used to build cell membranes, some *hormones*, and other important tissues and chemicals. The body can produce enough cholesterol on its own, so none is required in the diet. When people consume large amounts of cholesterol (found only in animal products), this can accelerate *atherosclerosis*.

claudication: Pain in the leg muscles caused by atherosclerotic narrowing of the *arteries* supplying blood to the legs. The pain usually starts during walking and subsides with rest.

coarctation of the aorta: A *congenital* condition in which the *aorta* is constricted. Coarctation of the aorta is a rare cause of *hypertension* in young children.

complicated hypertension: *Hypertension* in which there is evidence of organ damage related to *blood pressure*. Complications of hypertension include *stroke, congestive heart failure, kidney* failure, *heart attack,* and *aneurysm*.

computed tomography (CT) scanning: A diagnostic imaging technique in which a computer detects and analyzes X rays that are passed through the body from various angles to create cross-sectional pictures of a selected part of the body. Also called a CT scan, computed tomography gives doctors useful information about the structure and function of tissues and organs, including the *kidneys, arteries,* and heart.

congenital: A condition, especially an abnormality, that exists at birth. Congenital defects can be inherited (heredity) or caused by a problem during pregnancy.

congestive heart failure: A condition in which the heart cannot pump enough blood to meet the body's needs. Symptoms include shortness of breath, *edema,* and congestion in the lungs.

coronary: Refers to the heart.

coronary arteries: The *arteries* that supply oxygenated blood directly to the heart.

CT scanning: See *computed tomography (CT) scanning*.

Cushing's syndrome: A condition in which the *adrenal glands* produce too much of the *hormone* cortisol, which results in obesity, acne, purple streaks on the abdomen, and *hypertension*. Cushing's syndrome can be caused by a tumor in the adrenal gland.

D

diabetes: A disorder in which the body cannot properly maintain blood glucose (sugar) levels. The two main forms of the disease are type I (insulin-dependent) diabetes and type II (non–insulin-dependent) diabetes.

diastole: The period between heartbeats when the heart relaxes and fills with blood. See also *systole.*

diastolic blood pressure: The force of blood against the artery walls when the heart relaxes between beats. This is represented by the second number in a *blood pressure* reading. See also *systolic blood pressure.*

diuretic: A type of medication that helps the body to eliminate excess *sodium* and water, thus reducing *blood pressure.*

E

echocardiography: *Ultrasound scanning* of the heart, including its valves and inner chambers.

eclampsia: A life-threatening condition in which a pregnant woman with *preeclampsia* experiences seizures and possible coma.

edema: Any accumulation of fluid in the body, such as when the ankles swell because of heart failure, during pregnancy, or as the result of medication use.

electrocardiography: A procedure that records the electrical activity of the heart muscle through electrodes (small discs with wires attached) placed at specific locations on the chest and arms.

embolism: Obstruction of a blood vessel by an embolus (blood clot or air bubble).

endocrinologist: A doctor who specializes in treatment of disorders of the glands.

endothelium: The thin, delicate, inner lining of the blood vessels.

epinephrine: A *hormone* (also called adrenaline) produced by the *adrenal glands* that increases the heart rate and blood flow.

F

fibromuscular hyperplasia: A condition, usually found in young women, in which the walls of the *renal arteries* become constricted by extra muscle and fibrous tissue that hardens into rings. One symptom of this condition is *hypertension.*

free radicals: Substances produced by the body's normal processes that cause damage to cells and to the genetic material inside the cells.

This damage contributes to many disorders, including heart disease and cancer, and promotes aging.

G

gangrene: A condition in which body tissue dies because of a lack of blood. People with *diabetes* are at high risk for gangrene.

glomerulonephritis: A type of *kidney* disease in which the tiny filtering units of the kidneys are inflamed and unable to remove waste products from the blood.

H

heart attack: Death of part of the heart muscle caused by lack of blood supply. The medical term for heart attack is myocardial infarction.

high blood pressure: See *hypertension*.

hormone: A chemical messenger that is formed in one organ or tissue and circulates through the blood to have a specific effect on another organ or tissue. *Insulin* and *epinephrine* are two hormones that play a part in maintaining *blood pressure*.

hyperaldosteronism: A condition in which the *adrenal glands* produce too much *aldosterone*. *Hypertension* is one symptom of this condition.

hyperkalemia: An abnormally high level of *potassium* in the blood. The excess potassium can cause irregular heart rhythms.

hypertension: A condition (also called high *blood pressure*) in which blood pressure is consistently elevated (higher than 140/90 mm Hg in adults). Hypertension directly increases the risk of *heart attack*, *stroke*, and *kidney* failure.

hypokalemia: Abnormally low levels of *potassium* in the blood. Symptoms include muscle weakness, breathing difficulties, muscle twitches, and, if left untreated, *arrhythmia*.

hypotension: Abnormally low *blood pressure*. This is usually not a medical problem, but low blood pressure can sometimes cause light-headedness or fainting if the brain does not receive enough blood.

I

insulin: A *hormone* produced by the pancreas that is essential to the use of glucose (blood sugar) in the body.

insulin resistance syndrome: A condition in which certain tissues in the body resist the effects of *insulin*, allowing glucose levels to rise. One major symptom of this syndrome is *hypertension*.

ischemia: Reduced blood supply to an organ or tissue due to blockage or narrowing of an *artery*.

isolated systolic hypertension: A condition in which *systolic blood pressure* is 140 mm Hg or higher and *diastolic blood pressure* is 90 mm Hg or lower.

K

kidneys: The two organs that filter out unwanted material from the blood and regulate the *blood volume*. Disorders of the kidney can cause *hypertension*, and the kidneys are especially susceptible to damage caused by high *blood pressure*.

L

lipids: A group of substances that are vital to many important body functions. Fats, fatty acids, triglycerides, and *cholesterol* are all lipids.

M

magnetic resonance imaging (MRI): A diagnostic imaging technique that uses a powerful magnet, radio waves, and a computer to generate cross-sectional pictures of the body. MRI produces useful information about the structure and function of tissues and organs, including *arteries* and the beating heart, without exposing the person to any radiation.

malignant hypertension: A condition in which significantly elevated *blood pressure* is accompanied by specific visible damage to the blood vessels in the back of the eye. Malignant hypertension can damage the *kidneys,* brain, eyes, and heart and is usually fatal unless treated promptly and aggressively.

MRI: See *magnetic resonance imaging.*

myocardial infarction: See *heart attack.*

N

nephrons: The microscopic filtering units of the *kidneys*.

neurotransmitters: Chemicals released by nerve cells to communicate with other nerve cells or other tissues in the body. For example, *norepinephrine* released by nerve cells in the *sympathetic nervous system* directs blood vessels to constrict, raising *blood pressure*.

noradrenaline: See *norepinephrine*.

norepinephrine: A chemical released as a *neurotransmitter* by nerve cells (specifically in the *sympathetic nervous system*), and as a *hormone* by the *adrenal glands*, that raises *blood pressure* by constricting the *arteries* and increasing the heart rate.

O

orthostatic hypotension: See *postural hypotension*.

P

palpitation: An abnormally strong, rapid heartbeat.

peripheral resistance: The resistance of blood vessels to the flow of blood being pumped by the heart. Peripheral resistance is one of two forces responsible for *blood pressure* (the other is the pumping of the heart). When blood vessels constrict, peripheral resistance and blood pressure go up.

peripheral vascular disease: A narrowing of the blood vessels that limits blood flow to a specific part of the body (such as the hands, feet, or legs), causing numbness and pain.

pheochromocytoma: A tumor (usually noncancerous) of the *adrenal gland* that can cause excessive amounts of specific *hormones* to be produced, raising *blood pressure*.

placebo: A term used to describe empty or inactive treatment of any sort (such as sugar pills) that does not actually have any effect on the body but that may result in improvement because of the psychological state of the person receiving treatment. That is, if the person truly believes he or she is being treated, his or her brain might bring about the desired physical changes and improvement in health.

platelet: The smallest circulating blood cell, which is responsible for forming clots in response to both cuts in the skin and injury to the lining of the blood vessels. Platelets can also stimulate growth in certain tissues of the *arteries*, which is usually helpful but can contribute to the development of *atherosclerosis*.

polycystic kidney disease: An inherited condition in which multiple cysts of varying size develop in both *kidneys*, causing damage to the kidneys and *hypertension*.

postural hypotension: Abnormally low *blood pressure* that occurs in response to a sudden change in body position (from lying to sitting or from sitting to standing), which causes dizziness or fainting.

potassium: A mineral needed by the body for conduction of nerve impulses, contraction of muscles, proper functioning of enzymes, maintaining fluid balance, and sustaining a normal heart rhythm.

preeclampsia: A serious condition (also known as toxemia of pregnancy) in which a woman past her 20th week of pregnancy develops *hypertension* and *edema*. If untreated, this condition can lead to *eclampsia*.

prostaglandin: Hormonelike substances produced in the body that can increase *blood pressure* by constricting blood vessels.

proteinuria: Abnormally high levels of protein in the urine.

R

renal: Refers to the *kidneys*.

renin: An enzyme produced by the *kidneys* that helps regulate *blood pressure*.

renovascular hypertension: A condition in which *hypertension* is caused by a blockage in one or both of the *renal arteries*.

retina: The light-sensitive membrane lining the inside of the back of the eye. The *arteries* of the retina can be observed directly by shining a light on the retina, allowing your doctor to monitor the health of arteries throughout your body.

retinopathy: Damage to or disease of the *retina*, often caused by persistent *hypertension*.

S

salt: A chemical compound of *sodium* (40 percent) and chloride (60 percent).

sodium: A mineral in the cells of the body that is essential for maintaining *blood pressure,* fluid balance, proper conduction of nerve impulses, and muscle contraction.

sphygmomanometer: A device used to measure *blood pressure.*

stethoscope: A device used to listen to sounds inside the body.

stroke: Brain damage caused by interrupted blood flow to part of the brain. Stroke can occur when a blood vessel in the brain ruptures or is blocked (as by a blood clot). Possible symptoms include paralysis, loss of sensation, and loss of consciousness. The damage may or may not be permanent. See also *transient ischemic attack (TIA).*

sympathetic nervous system: The part of the *autonomic nervous system* that increases the heart rate and raises *blood pressure.*

systole: The period during the heartbeat when the heart contracts and pumps blood out to the tissues. See also *diastole.*

systolic blood pressure: The force of blood against the artery walls when the heart contracts and pumps blood out to the tissues. This is represented by the first number in a *blood pressure* reading. See also *diastolic blood pressure.*

T

thrombosis: Formation of a blood clot inside a blood vessel.

transient ischemic attack (TIA): Temporary interruption of the blood supply to the brain, which causes *stroke*like symptoms (such as weakness, difficulty speaking, and numbness) that last for a few minutes up to several hours. A TIA occurs when a small piece of atherosclerotic plaque breaks loose and temporarily blocks an artery in the brain.

U

ultrasound scanning: A diagnostic imaging technique that uses high-frequency sound waves and a computer to generate pictures of organs and tissues inside the body. Ultrasound examination provides valuable information about the structure and function of such organs as the heart and *kidneys.*

uremia: A condition in which *kidney* failure causes waste products to accumulate in the blood.

V

vascular: Refers to blood vessels (*arteries, veins,* and *capillaries*).

vasoconstrictor: A chemical (drug, *neurotransmitter,* or *hormone*) that causes blood vessels to constrict (tighten).

vasodilator: A chemical (drug, *neurotransmitter,* or *hormone*) that causes blood vessels to dilate (widen).

vein: A blood vessel that carries deoxygenated blood from the body tissues back to the heart. The only exceptions are the pulmonary veins, which carry oxygenated blood from the lungs to the heart.

W

white-coat hypertension: A condition in which a person's *blood pressure* rises in clinical settings, such as at the doctor's office, at a public health screening, or whenever a health-care professional measures blood pressure.

Index

Please note: Medications are indexed by generic name only.